A Nutritional Healing guide
By Lynn Marie Jackson
2025

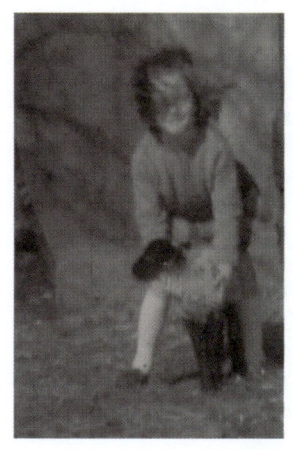 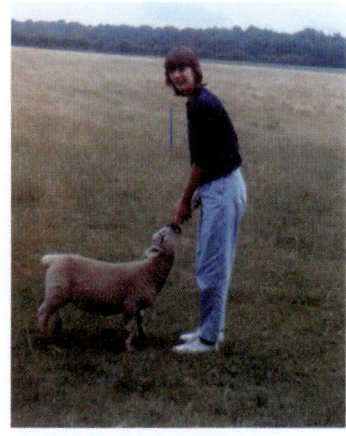

**For my mum
Enid**

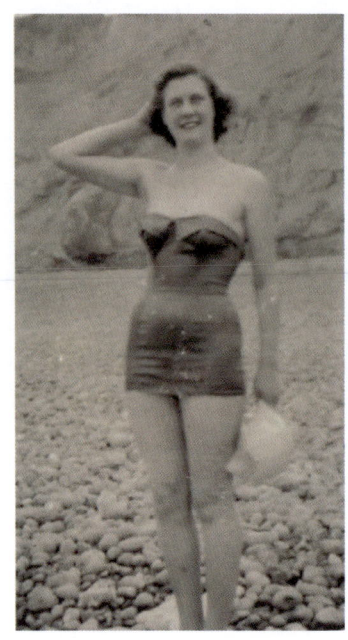

Disclaimer

The information provided in this book is intended as general guidance for individuals seeking a holistic approach to healing. It is NOT a substitute for professional medical care, pharmaceutical treatments, or advice from your doctor or healthcare provider.

Before making any changes to your medications, diet, or health routines, consult with your NHS doctor or qualified medical professional. If you are considering adjusting or discontinuing any prescribed medications, seek medical supervision to ensure your safety and well-being.

Nutritional and lifestyle changes should complement—not replace—medical treatments and interventions. Regular check-ups and blood tests with your healthcare provider are essential to monitor and manage any health conditions or concerns.

Healing and healthy living work best when integrated with professional medical advice and care.

" The nutritional Healer " can be found 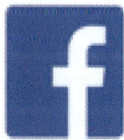  @

@All rights reserved Norfolk

No copies or digital sharing of this book is allowed without the sole authorisation of the author.

Introduction.

I was born on a small sheep farm in Norfolk, UK, in 1963, the youngest of four children—two boys and two girls. My childhood was a mix of fresh air, healthy food, and hard work. My mother always ensured we had good meals on the table, but by the time I was eight, things started to change. Her health began to deteriorate, and she was told her conditions were genetic. She accepted the diagnoses, relied on medications, and over the years ended up taking 29 pills and two daily injections. Despite her stoic nature, watching her suffer was upsetting. She lived her life with incredible strength but passed away after 47 years of struggle.

Growing up, I tried not to add to my mother's worries. I supported her by helping out, from feeding lambs in the barn to helping in the garden, decorating the home, and managing chores. I also worked alongside my father, doing everything from helping with the shearing of sheep, by penning them up and rolling up the wool. To dipping them and running them through foot baths, to walking them along roads to new fields to graze on sugar beet tops, carrots, and cabbages during the winter months. My most important job was looking after orphaned lambs, which could be sad at times.

Farm life was tough, but it was all I knew. My father once told me that my lambs he sold at the market went to live in an orchard with a kind old lady he had met, where they would graze happily until they passed from old age. I realised this was a fairy story and he smiled, but stories are important sometimes to keep moral up. Outside of farm duties, I had a busy, adventure-filled childhood, exploring rivers, collecting chestnuts, building huts, and riding bikes with my siblings and the farm over the roads children. The countryside was our adventure playground.

Thanks to my mother being able to drive and her father's generosity in gifting her old cars, we often went to the beach. Those seaside trips were a cherished escape from daily chores, filled with laughter and play.

However, by the age of ten, I began experiencing health issues—gut problems, asthma, eczema, and dizziness (now known as POTS). In my late teens, stress took a toll when my sister fell seriously ill, and I soon followed. By my twenties, I had several diagnoses and was on various medications, which only made me feel a whole lot worse. Without the internet, there was no way of researching or challenge all what I was told. I assumed I was simply unlucky, despite eating better than most people I knew. So, I naturally assumed my diet should be good enough and it must be as they said a genetic fault.

It wasn't until decades later that I stumbled upon a different narrative. Determined to find answers, I dived into researching, exploring diet and health in depth. The journey was overwhelming at first—there was so much conflicting information. I experimented with different approaches, gradually piecing together a plan that worked for me. Slowly, over 14 months of hard work, my health improved. Weaning off medications was another 6 month battle. Doctors had warned me that I'd needed them for life, but I was resolute. Over the months, I used diet, through Christmas, birthdays and outings and stuck religiously to my plan, yoga, and walking to rebuild my health. Then, over another six months, I tackled withdrawal symptoms and finally became medication-free. Ten years later, I remain healthy and unmedicated to this day.

Inspired by my own journey, I pursued training in nutrition, gut health, brain health, and naturopathy, including herbalism. I read countless scientific papers and found joy in learning and finding answers my doctors had failed to provide for me and others.

I decided to write a book with everything I had learnt, to help others find the answers they wished for and design healing paths. What I had managed to do alone, I thought it would be nice to have a plan for others to follow, to make it easier than my journey. I hope this book provides the answers you have been looking for and inspires you to not believe all we are told and realise our minds and bodies abilities to heal are far greater than anyone on this planet has ever permitted us to believe in. This ancient healing was all but lost, but many like me are finding it and managing to turn around all that science and research said we couldn't. It nice to prove "experts" wrong sometimes, it gives us a little smile.

Forward.
If you are struggling with ill health and seeking ways to support your body and achieve healing, you've picked up the right book. Inside these pages, you'll find detailed chapters on a variety of health conditions, including autoimmune diseases like lupus and thyroid disorders, mental health issues such as depression, bipolar disorder, and schizophrenia, as well as ADHD and autism. For each condition, I've included protocols tailored to support healing, backed by scientific studies I've uncovered on PubMed and other reputable sources. While some of the science remains inconclusive, it often provides valuable insights, helping us focus on practical steps for recovery.

A key theme throughout this book is the understanding that health conditions often stem from multiple causes. It's important to differentiate between a trigger and the underlying causes of an illness. Triggers may set off a condition, but most health issues have multiple drivers—whether it's inflammation, gut imbalances, or environmental factors. As a result, the protocols I've designed address a wide range of potential causes. They take a holistic approach, ensuring that all contributing factors are covered, so you can begin healing regardless of the root cause.

For instance, inflammation is a common driver behind many illnesses. I'll guide you through what an anti-inflammatory diet looks like and help you understand the mechanisms behind inflammation—why it happens and how to reverse it. Conditions like acid reflux (a gut issue), high blood pressure (a blood issue), and high cholesterol (a liver issue) often share similar underlying causes, so the protocols overlap in many areas. Mental health conditions, for example, may be rooted in stress, trauma, or inflammation of the nervous system—often tied to gut health, as the majority of serotonin is produced in the gut. To address this, I've included strategies to calm the adrenals, reduce cortisol levels, and heal gut dysbiosis, which is common in conditions like IBS and celiac disease.

Behind many chronic conditions lie bacteria, pathogens, or imbalances in the microbiome, which require targeted protocols. The plans I provide are comprehensive, addressing everything the body needs daily to heal. Unlike general advice to "eat healthily" or follow moderation, these protocols are specifically tailored to bring chronic conditions into remission. Healing takes commitment and effort, and these strategies aim to give you a clear, actionable plan to achieve results.

For those on medication, it's possible to work toward reducing or even eliminating them under the guidance of your doctor. Conditions like type 2 diabetes, for example, can improve to the point where medications can be reduced gradually, based on blood test results. But the first step is nutritional work. This book provides the tools you need to achieve remission and even reversal of many common illnesses, including autoimmune diseases. These approaches are inspired by the work of functional medicine doctors and my personal experience.

I also address the role of supplements—what genuinely helps and what's more of a gimmick. If supplements are beyond your budget, don't worry—everything can be achieved through diet alone. You'll find healing recipes, juices, and smoothies throughout this book to support your journey.

Healing takes time and effort, but results will come if you stay consistent. Progress doesn't require perfection; it simply requires a willingness to start and stick with it. My own journey was full of challenges, but I kept learning, adapting, and improving. Over time, I created recipes and strategies that turned healing into an enjoyable process.

Lastly, I focus on health, not weight loss. The advice to "exercise more and eat less" is often ineffective—it leads to hunger and frustration. Instead, this book emphasizes nourishing your body with sufficient, satisfying food. Forget calorie counting; what matters is the quality of the food you eat and how it supports your body's healing.

Remember, healing is a journey. Take it one step at a time, and trust that your efforts will be rewarded. This book is your guide to reclaiming your health and finding a path to lasting wellness.

Contents	page number
Introduction	6
forward	7
How we become **chronically ill...toxicities, chemicals, pathogens and stress**	9
Healing the gut	11
All about auto immune dis eases...**lupus and rheumatoid arthritis** etc	15
All about **mental health...depression and bipolar** etc	16
All about **autism and ADHD** etc	21
All about **Alzheimer's and dementia and Parkinson's** etc	25
All about **diabetes and the gall bladder**	28
All about **high blood pressure and high cholesterol** etc	30
All about **menopause, endometriosis, fibroids and PCOS** etc	35
All about **Crohn's and colitis and IBD and celiac** etc	39
All about **asthma and eczema and allergies**	42
All about **herbs and roots and spices**	46
All about **long covid and chronic fatigue syndrome and fibromyalgia**	47
All about the **KETO diet, the low carb diet and neurological inflammation**	52
All about troublesome foods and drinks	54
Juicers and blenders	56
Breakfasts, juices, smoothies and herbal teas etc	57
Lunches and salads and soups	65
Tea and traybakes and hot pots	71
Acid and alkaline balance	78
Snacks and sweet treats and puddings	79
Daily healing protocols for all chronic health dis eases	84
List of chronic conditions and their root causes/drivers	88
A Nutritional healing Guide to Reclaiming Your Health	90
Sound healing frequencies to listen to	92
References	93
Colds and flu	94
Immunity boosting broth	95

How We Become Chronically Ill: Toxicities, Chemicals, Pathogens, and Stress
Chronic illness often results from a combination of factors that strain our immune systems. These include genetics, cultural habits, environmental exposures, pathogens, parasites, and toxic substances. Stress, along with inadequate rest and relaxation, plays a significant role, as do the effects of trauma and abuse that some individuals—especially children—endure. The modern world has become an increasingly toxic environment for humans, with countless contributors to poor health building up over time. Eventually, this toxic load can overwhelm our immune systems. However, understanding how our bodies function and naturally cleanse themselves allows us to support these vital detoxification pathways. By eliminating poisons, gently cleansing our organs, repairing the gut microbiome, and detoxifying the lymphatic system, we can initiate deep healing. These practices tap into ancient knowledge—once widely understood and utilized but now nearly lost or hidden.

Historically, women often held this healing wisdom, using their understanding of nature's remedies to care for the sick and dying. Unfortunately, this knowledge was suppressed over time. Women who practiced healing were labelled as "witches," persecuted, and punished, leading to fear and silence. Many stopped sharing their healing practices altogether, while others continued in secrecy to avoid persecution. This silencing of traditional healing knowledge has left a void in our understanding of how to work with nature to restore health.

Today, chronic illness is often driven by inflammation and oxidative stress, alongside toxicities, pathogens, and parasites such as viruses, bacteria, fungi, Mold, and yeasts. These root causes have always been at the heart of disease. Yet modern healthcare, as a highly profitable industry, often focuses on symptom suppression rather than addressing the underlying causes. Patients are encouraged to rely on medications while being promised future cures, contingent on more funding for research.

Meanwhile, some individuals have managed to heal themselves by returning to this lost wisdom, supporting their bodies' natural processes, and addressing the real drivers of disease. Healing is possible, even in a world where the system often fails to provide true solutions.

Inflammation and Oxidative Stress: Hidden Drivers of Illness
Inflammation and oxidative stress are natural processes that, when uncontrolled, contribute to chronic illnesses like heart disease, diabetes, and mental health disorders.

Inflammation is the body's defence against injury or infection. While acute inflammation heals damage, chronic inflammation, often caused by poor diet, stress, or toxins, persists and harms tissues and organs. It's also linked to gut imbalances, which can trigger systemic inflammation and even mental health issues.

Oxidative stress occurs when free radicals—unstable molecules—overwhelm antioxidants, leading to cell damage. Factors like pollution, smoking, and poor diet worsen oxidative stress, which accelerates aging and drives diseases like Alzheimer's and cancer.

These two processes fuel each other, creating a harmful cycle. For example, in heart disease, oxidative stress damages blood vessels, triggering inflammation that worsens the condition.

Breaking this cycle requires an anti-inflammatory diet rich in fruits, vegetables, and healthy fats, along with antioxidants like vitamin C. Lifestyle changes such as managing stress, exercising, and improving sleep also help reduce inflammation and oxidative stress.

By addressing these factors, we can restore balance, lower disease risk, and support overall health.

I am Witch [healer] ... A poem....

A witch is a wise woman, a healer, a wortcunner (herbalist), a grandmother, a bonesetter, a mid-wife. She is a cunning woman — one who knows. She is a woman who understands the powers of the changing seasons and the phases of celestial bodies. She is the woman in your village who will come to your home when you are ailing with a cauldron of herbal tea and sit with her loving and healing hand on your back while you drink it. A witch is part shaman, part psychologist. She understands not only how to choose the right root for the cure, but what must be healed at the root to make a person whole: a broken heart; an angry liver; lungs full of grief; etc.

These women honed their wisdom and craft not through some dark sorcery, but through quiet lives filled with careful study and communion with the natural world, and they passed down their wisdom in lineages that spanned millennia. Witches not only facilitated wellness and healing, they advised and assisted in all aspects of life effected by the Turning of the Seasonal Wheel. They knew the right time to plant a seed and the particular moment to cut a leaf or harvest a root for optimum potency. They were effective, humble, and dedicated servants of their communities. And what did they receive for this service? Gratitude? Accolades? Tragically, no. For their service to humanity these wise healing women were killed by the millions. They were tortured on racks, eviscerated, drawn and quartered, burned at the stake, boiled alive in pots, and drowned in rivers and in barrels. They were raped and defiled in ways no one should ever have to think about never mind experience. When they hung these poor women, they did so with a short rope because it was not enough just to kill them, they had to torture them first, and a short rope does not snap the neck, it strangles. This is patriarchy; this is femicide; this is the destruction of the living legacy of the power of women at its most diabolical. And the more powerful these women were, the more successful their healing graces, the better they served their communities, the greater the chance that they would be taken to the slaughter because success was seen as proof that they must have powers that "come from the devil." When things went wrong, they were also blamed. When a child failed to thrive, a cow quit giving milk, or when a person died despite the best efforts of a healing woman, people in their grief (and need for a scapegoat), and powerful men looking for an excuse to take them down, went after these women often burning their homes and taking their lives. And that, is true evil, to use superstition and fear to crush powerful women to dust.

Because, even to this day, a powerful woman, standing in her wisdom and strength is something that many will simply not abide. As religions grew in power and as a male-only chemical based medical system came into dominance, the demonization and slaughter of these wortcunners, midwives and village healers became a genocide. So many died we will never know the full numbers. Because of their "evil" most were dumped in pauper's graves and their families were left to mourn in isolation. But today the goddess is rising, and we witches are rising strong with her. Today women are beginning to come back to their rightful places of power and with them they bring circles instead of hierarchies. They bring not only cures, but deep healing. For in our creative and generative power, women stand in symbol and purpose as Mother Nature to all living things on our planet. I pray each day that together we guide a better world into being.

Today herbal medicine, methods of hands-on healing, biodynamic and organic farming —all the realms of witches— are becoming widespread again and women are leading the way. But you may ask, What of magick? Aren't witches magick? And the answer is, yes! Yes we are. Because magick is just another form of mindfulness. To know how to be still, to meditate, to listen to messages spoken by the wind, to hear the voice of a tender spring shoot, to feel the pulse and rhythm of life at its deepest levels: this is the magick of the witch. This is my magick and I feel it running deep in my courage bones every moment of my life. So, I stand proudly before you today and every day of my life on the graves of my slaughtered sisters to take back this word, witch. To retrieve it from its place as hate speech, and elevate it to a word of power in its true meaning. I stand up to honour them and in order to make sure that hate, fear and patriarchy never again try to wipe us from the face of the earth.

Healing the Gut: The Foundation of Wellness

Healing the gut is essential for overall health. For those with sensitive digestion, it's important to start slowly. Avoiding too many raw salads initially and focusing on soothing, easy-to-digest foods like smoothies, soups, fruits, coconut oil, and bone broth. Triggers such as dairy, eggs, grains, coffee, fizzy drinks, sugar, and processed foods should be eliminated.

Transitioning to a gut-healing plan takes time, especially for individuals with inflamed or sensitive stomachs. Progress at your own pace—there's no race to healing. Rushing can stress the body, so steady, gradual changes are key.

One common issue to address is "leaky gut syndrome," a condition where weak intestinal lining allows gases and tiny food particles to pass through, triggering an immune response. This can lead to symptoms like histamine intolerance, allergies, migraines, and inflammation.

By healing the gut, we can alleviate symptoms of autoimmune diseases and conditions such as skin problems, asthma, hormonal imbalances, chronic fatigue, brain fog, mood swings, and digestive discomforts like cramps, bloating, and IBS. A calm, healthy gut is the foundation for a vibrant body and mind.

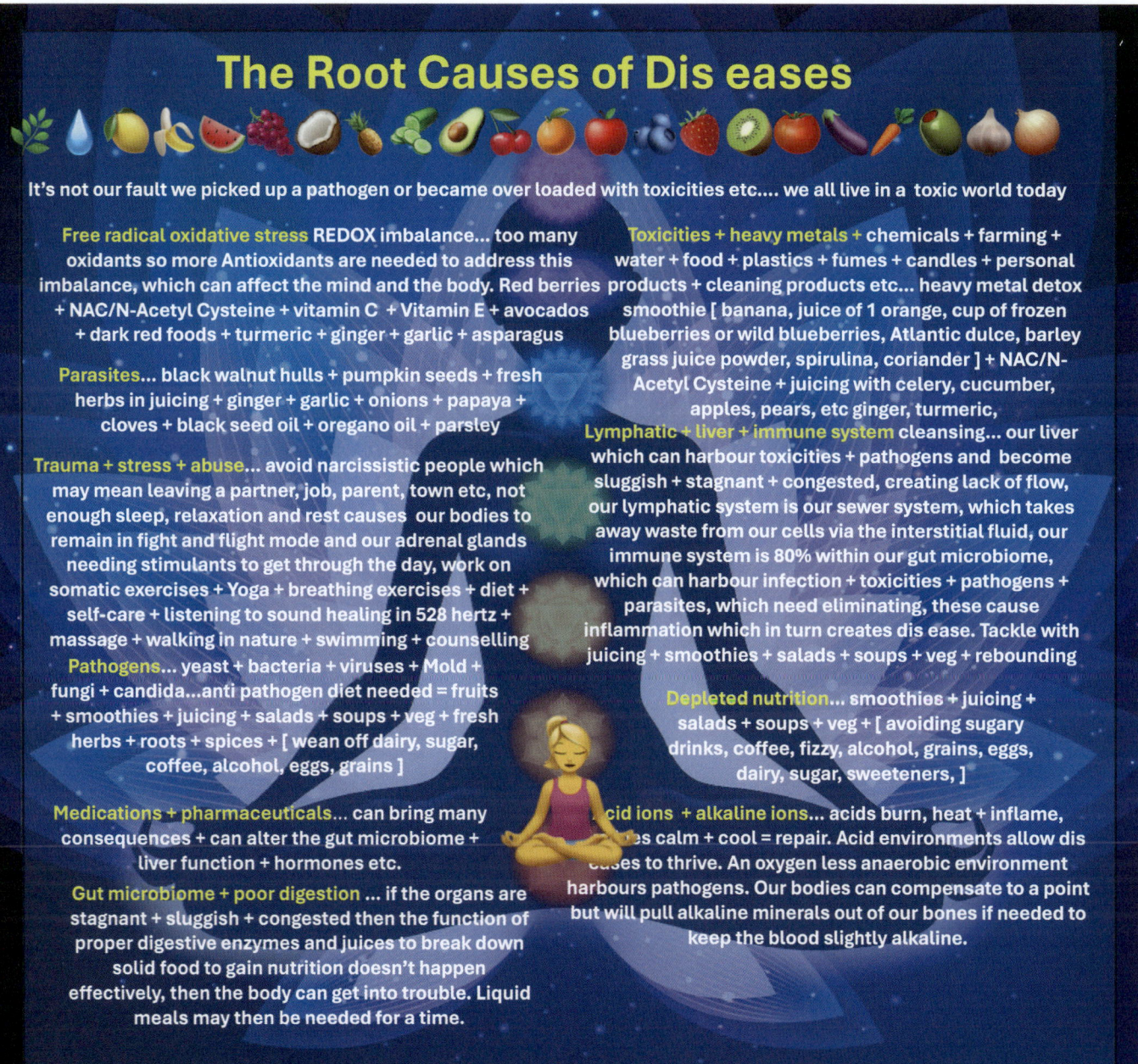

The Root Causes of Dis eases

1 Free radical oxidative stress REDOX imbalance... too many oxidants so more Antioxidants are needed to address this imbalance, which can affect the mind and the body. Red berries + NAC/N-Acetyl Cysteine + vitamin C + Vitamin E + avocados + dark red foods + turmeric + ginger + garlic + asparagus + leafy greens + fresh herbs + spices.

2 Toxicities + heavy metals + chemicals + farming + water + food + plastics + fumes + candles + personal products + cleaning products etc... heavy metal detox smoothie [banana, juice of 1 orange, cup of frozen blueberries or wild blueberries, Atlantic dulce, barley grass juice powder, spirulina, coriander] + NAC/N-Acetyl Cysteine + juicing with celery, cucumber, apples, pears, etc ginger, turmeric.

3 Lymphatic + liver + immune system cleansing... our liver which can harbour toxicities + pathogens and become sluggish + stagnant + congested, creating lack of flow, our lymphatic system is our sewer system, which takes away waste from our cells via the interstitial fluid, our immune system is 80% within our gut microbiome, which can harbour infection + toxicities + pathogens + parasites, which need eliminating, these cause inflammation which in turn creates dis ease. Tackle with juicing + smoothies + salads + soups + veg + rebounding.

4 Trauma + stress + abuse... avoid narcissistic people which may mean leaving a partner, job, parent, town etc, not enough sleep, relaxation and rest causes our bodies to remain in fight and flight mode and our adrenal glands needing stimulants to get through the day, work on somatic exercises + Yoga + breathing exercises + diet + self-care + listening to sound healing in 528 hertz + massage + walking in nature + swimming + counselling.

5 Pathogens... yeast + bacteria + viruses + Mold + fungi + candida...anti pathogen diet needed = fruits + smoothies + juicing + salads + soups + veg + fresh herbs + roots + spices + [wean off dairy, sugar, coffee, alcohol, eggs, grains]

6 Acid ions + alkaline ions... acids burn, heat + inflame, alkalines calm + cool = repair. Acid environments allow dis eases to thrive. An oxygen less anaerobic environment harbours pathogens. Our bodies can compensate to a point but will pull alkaline minerals out of our bones if needed to keep the blood slightly alkaline.

7 Gut microbiome + poor digestion ... if the organs are stagnant + sluggish + congested then the function of proper digestive enzymes and juices to break down solid food to gain nutrition doesn't happen effectively, then the body can get into trouble. Liquid meals may then be needed for a time.

8 Depleted nutrition... smoothies + juicing + salads + soups + veg + [avoiding sugary drinks, coffee, fizzy, alcohol, grains, eggs, dairy, sugar, sweeteners,]

9 Parasites... black walnut hulls + pumpkin seeds + fresh herbs in juicing + ginger + garlic + onions + papaya + cloves + black seed oil + oregano oil + parsley

10 Medications + pharmaceuticals + treatments... can bring many consequences + they can alter the gut microbiome + liver function + hormones etc. [long term]

So, as you can see, there are many different complexed reasons as to why we become ill. It's not solely our own fault, as we all now live in a super toxic world and once our bodies and minds become overloaded with these toxic things, our health can slide greatly. Also, the treatments that have short term gains, can also come with long term harms. The use of too many anti biotics can harm our gut microbiome and in turn weaken our immune systems, making us vulnerable to other illnesses and chronic conditions. Healing is the undoing of all these things using natural means, as in mother nature. This should be used alongside western allopathic medical treatments and not in place of. When ill, we must try and do everything in our power to regain and restore our health. Sadly, this doesn't always happen amongst all the confusions, many people can and do get lost on the path.

Healing in a Toxic World
Our bodies are designed to be self-cleansing, but in today's world, the toxic load has surpassed what many sensitive individuals can handle. These people, often referred to as "the canaries in the coal mine," are the first to signal the dangers of our environment.

Mental and neurological health is under unprecedented threat. Never before have so many people, across all ages, struggled with conditions like epilepsy, autism, dementia, Alzheimer's, ADHD, ALS, functional neurological disease, and Parkinson's. Many of these conditions are linked to toxins and chemicals that disrupt our bodily systems, interfering with electrical signals and causing malfunctions.

Fortunately, there is much we can do. By cleansing the body and supporting the liver and lymphatic systems, we can help eliminate these toxic invaders. There are numerous natural strategies, herbs, and foods that can be incorporated into daily life to aid this process. This journey—our healing journey—requires a daily commitment to support the mind and body in their recovery.

The healing journey
Healing is not about finding a magic herb or miracle meal. It's about consistency, persistence, and the willingness to adopt new habits while letting go of old, unhelpful ones. Many of these attachments stem from childhood, culture, or parental habits. The healing process involves releasing what no longer serves us and embracing practices that promote health.

Everyone's journey is different. Some may face mild illness lasting a few months, while others may have decades of chronic conditions and even be bedridden. The level of effort required depends on the individual, but one thing is certain: it is never too late to try. The fear that it's "too late" can stop people from starting, but the body is far more remarkable than we often realize.

Turning things around requires courage and a desire for change. Healing is hard work and may involve suffering along the way, but the reward of overcoming autoimmune diseases or chronic mental health conditions is worth the effort. The journey, though challenging, becomes meaningful when we reach our goal.

The Role of Faith and Action
There are no guarantees in life, but doing nothing guarantees nothing. Healing requires self-work and commitment. Once we achieve recovery, we can share our stories with those who are ready to heal. While many people need healing, not everyone is ready to embark on this journey. All we can do is share our experiences and show kindness to those we encounter.

Scepticism is natural, especially when people share their personal stories without scientific proof. Many continue to wait for medical science to deliver cures, raising money and placing faith in future research. While waiting, some may try various diets, fads, or advice from books and experts, only to feel lost and overwhelmed.

I was once like this—waiting, wishing, and feeling powerless. Before the internet, information was scarce, and now we face the opposite problem: an overwhelming flood of paths and choices. Many people flit from one diet or fad to another without fully understanding what healing truly involves.

A Clear Path Forward
This book is meant to provide clarity. I will share everything I've learned so you can have a clear, actionable path to follow. With the right guidance and protocols, you can embark on your healing journey with confidence and purpose.

The Myth of a Single Cause and Cure

Science and research often focus immense time and money looking backward, searching for "the" cause of a disease. The hope is that uncovering a single cause will lead to "the" cure. However, our bodies don't work like that. There was, and never will be, just one cause for most illnesses. While there may be a final trigger—like the proverbial straw that breaks the camel's back—illness is usually the result of many causes, unique to each individual.

Even two people with the same diagnosis, such as lupus, may have completely different sets of causes or, as I call them, "drivers." This is why a universal "cure-all" medication is an impossibility. Thinking of illness in such simplistic terms is unhelpful and even foolish.

Forward Thinking in Healing

Instead of looking backward, trying to analyse every event that contributed to illness, we need to focus on the present. The healing practices in this book are rooted in forward thinking—learning and improving every day without dwelling on yesterday. Healing isn't about wishing our-selves well; it's about doing and being well. Praying without action is merely wishful thinking.

We often believe that if we think more, we'll understand more, and that understanding will lead to action. But true healing isn't a mental exercise. It requires stepping out of our thoughts and into our bodies. The body holds the answers. It communicates its needs if we are willing to listen and ask: *What does my body need? What choices can I make to support it better?*

The body cannot be tricked. Our immune systems and the innate intelligence of our design are far greater than human thought can fully comprehend. Our bodies were designed perfectly. When health falters, we must rise to the occasion and climb back to wellness—not by overthinking but by aligning with the body's wisdom.

The Sacred Path of Healing

For some, the healing journey is one they are forced onto—often out of desperation or the severity of illness. Sometimes it takes reaching stage four disease, or another crisis point before we awaken to what is necessary. These moments of reckoning can be painful and soul-searching. We may wrestle with blame, regret, or the narratives we've created to cope. But true healing demands courage.

Avoidance is easy. We can pass the metaphorical sword of healing down the family line, labelling the problem as "genetic" and leaving it for another soul to confront. Yet all healing is, in essence, ancestral. When someone in a lineage finally takes up the sword and succeeds in healing, they heal not just themselves but all those who come after them.

These are the sacred souls—the ones who break the chain, who undertake the long-lost and often misunderstood art of healing. Perhaps you are that soul. Perhaps you have stumbled upon these words because you are ready to take up the sword.

If so, I welcome you. Healing is always possible. It requires bravery, commitment, and an open mind. My aim is to guide you with simplicity and clarity, making this journey as accessible as possible.

Welcome to the healing path. There is much to learn, but you are not alone.

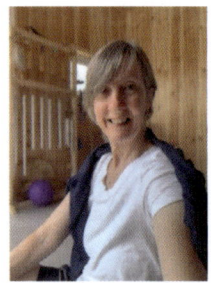

All about auto immune dis eases...lupus and rheumatoid arthritis [there are 11,702 science papers to read on pubmed.com about auto immune diseases]

Understanding Autoimmune Diseases: Causes, Triggers, and Healing

Autoimmune diseases are a vast category of over 100 conditions, including lupus, rheumatoid arthritis, multiple sclerosis, fibromyalgia, chronic fatigue syndrome (CFS/ME), celiac disease, Sjogren's syndrome, Crohn's disease, ulcerative colitis, endometriosis, long COVID, and many more. There are currently over 11,700 scientific papers on PubMed.com exploring autoimmune diseases, highlighting the complexity of these conditions.

The Root Causes of Autoimmune Diseases

Autoimmune conditions are not random malfunctions of the body; they are responses to underlying issues, including:

Pathogens & Viruses – Chronic infections, such as Epstein-Barr virus (EBV), Lyme disease, and herpes viruses, can trigger autoimmune responses.

Toxicity & Heavy Metals – Environmental pollutants, pesticides, Mold, and heavy metals (mercury, aluminium, lead) can disrupt immune function.

Gut Dysbiosis & Leaky Gut – A damaged gut lining allows toxins and undigested proteins to enter the bloodstream, leading to chronic inflammation.

Oxidative Stress & Redox Imbalance – A lack of antioxidants and an excess of free radicals contribute to cell damage and immune dysfunction.

Chronic Inflammation & Stress – High cortisol levels from prolonged stress weaken immune regulation and fuel disease progression.

The body does not attack itself without reason—there are always underlying drivers. These differ from person to person, making individualized healing strategies essential.

Steps to Healing: Addressing the Root Causes

Reversing or putting autoimmune diseases into remission requires a multi-faceted approach:

Pathogen & Toxicity Cleansing

Support detoxification with targeted herbs, binders, and liver-supporting foods.
Reduce exposure to environmental toxins, pesticides, and heavy metals.

Gut Repair & Anti-Inflammatory Nutrition

Restore the gut lining by eliminating inflammatory foods and incorporating gut-healing nutrients.
Follow an anti-inflammatory, nutrient-dense diet rich in whole foods.

Reducing Inflammatory Triggers

Gradually remove foods that fuel pathogens and inflammation, including:
Dairy, eggs, grains, refined sugar, artificial sweeteners, coffee, black tea, alcohol, processed foods, fermented foods, MSG, GMOs, preservatives, and vinegar.
This process takes time, patience, and commitment.

1. **Regulating Stress & Cortisol Levels**
   - Implement stress-reducing practices such as meditation, breathwork, and nature exposure.
   - Prioritize sleep and relaxation to allow the body to heal.

By addressing the root causes—pathogens, toxins, gut health, and inflammation—the body can restore balance and regain health. Healing is a journey, but with the right plan, many have reversed or put their autoimmune conditions into remission.

The Daily Cleansing choices + Healing Protocol

Nourishing & Healing Foods

Incorporating healing foods and drinks into your daily routine can support detoxification, reduce inflammation, and provide essential nutrients for overall well-being. Below are some powerful options:

Healing Drinks

Lemon or Ginger Water – Start your day with warm lemon or ginger-infused water to support digestion and detoxification.

Herbal Teas – Choose real herbal teas like thyme, chamomile, or peppermint. Add real honey or maple syrup for extra nourishment.

Celery Juice – Begin with ½ cup daily, gradually increasing to 1 pint per day over two weeks to support digestion, gut health, and detoxification.

Fresh Juice Blend – Juice together:

5 carrots
2 oranges
1 tsp real turmeric
1-inch piece of fresh ginger

Heavy Metal Detox Smoothie

A nutrient-dense smoothie designed to help remove heavy metals from the body:

1 cup blueberries
1–2 bananas
Juice of 1–2 oranges
½ cup fresh coriander
1 tsp spirulina
1 tsp Atlantic dulse
1 tsp barley grass juice powder

Wholesome Meals & Snacks

Salads – Combine avocado, leafy greens, asparagus, garlic, and other fresh vegetables. Dress with homemade dressing.

Roasted Vegetable Soup – Butternut squash, sweet potatoes, and seasonal vegetables blended into a warming soup.

Medjool Dates & Coconut Water – A great natural energy boost.

Lynn's Homemade Hot Chocolate – Blend together:

1 Medjool date
1 tsp gluten-free oats
1 square of 85% dark chocolate
Water
Cinnamon
Real maple syrup or honey

Homemade Treats

Lynn's Flapjacks – Made with gluten-free oats, maple syrup or honey, Medjool dates, and dark chocolate.

Lynn's Fruit Crumble – A wholesome, naturally sweetened dessert.

Key Healing Ingredients

Hot Pots, Tray Bakes, Soups, Salads, Juices, Smoothies – Incorporate a variety of fresh, organic ingredients daily.

Fruits & Vegetables – Prioritize fresh, nutrient-dense produce.
- **Fresh Herbs & Spices** – Use ginger, garlic, turmeric, cinnamon, cloves, and nutmeg for their anti-inflammatory benefits.
- **Healthy Fats** – Include coconut oil and olive oil for essential fatty acids and brain health.

Cleansing & Supporting the Lymphatic System

Our lymphatic system is the body's natural sewer system, responsible for clearing out toxins, pathogens, and waste. However, it can become stagnant, congested, and sluggish, leading to toxin buildup and inflammation. Supporting the lymphatic system is essential for overall health and immune function.

How to Cleanse & Detox the Lymphatic System

Juicing with Fresh Herbs – Parsley, cilantro, mint, and dandelion help flush toxins.
Green Detox Smoothies – Blending leafy greens, spirulina, barley grass, and chlorella helps remove heavy metals.
Alkaline Foods & Drinks – Raw fruits, vegetables, lemon water, and herbal teas support cellular cleansing.
Hydration – Pure water, coconut water, and hydrating herbal teas keep the lymph moving.
Movement – Rebounding, dry brushing, and sweating through exercise or saunas help stimulate lymph flow.

Restoring Gut & Immune Health

Since 80% of the immune system resides in the gut microbiome, detoxifying the lymph also benefits digestion, liver function, and adrenal health.
Cleansing the Liver & Lymph – Bitter greens, turmeric, beet juice, and celery juice support liver detox.
Calming the Adrenals & Kidneys – Adaptogenic herbs, hydration, and stress reduction lower cortisol and restore balance.

Fighting Pathogens & Reducing Inflammation

All fresh herbs, spices, and roots are naturally anti-pathogenic, antiviral, and antibacterial, helping to clear out harmful microbes.
Juicing & Smoothies with Green Detox Powders – Over time, these assist in chelating toxins and removing heavy metals.
Combatting Inflammation – Inflammation is the body's response to toxins, pathogens, and oxidative stress. A nutrient-dense, raw alkaline diet rich in antioxidants helps neutralize free radicals and restore REDOX balance (the equilibrium between free radicals and antioxidants).

By nourishing the body with the right foods, hydration, and lifestyle choices, you can restore lymphatic flow, detoxify the body, and reduce inflammation naturally.

HEALING + SUPPLEMENTS

Holistic Healing & Wellness Practices

True healing involves a combination of nutrition, detoxification, movement, relaxation, and emotional well-being. A multi-faceted approach can support the immune system, reduce inflammation, restore balance, and promote overall vitality.

1. Nutrition & Detoxification

Healing Foods – Juices, smoothies, salads, soups, fresh vegetables, and nutrient-dense whole foods.

Superfoods & Supplements:
Essential Vitamins & Minerals – Vitamin C, D, B12, zinc, omega-3 oils.
Detoxifiers – Spirulina, barley grass juice powder, Atlantic dulse, goldenseal, chaga mushrooms.
Herbs & Roots – Turmeric, ginger, garlic, cat's claw, echinacea, elderberry.
Liver & Gut Support – Milk thistle, blackstrap molasses, digestive enzymes, probiotics, prebiotics.
Immune & Cellular Support – NAC (N-acetyl cysteine), L-lysine, GABA, CoQ10, glutathione, astaxanthin.
Adaptogens & Healing Oils – Ashwagandha, CBD oil, black seed oil, oregano oil, kelp, ginseng, liquorice.
Detox Aids – Black walnut hulls, hibiscus, chamomile, rose hip, lemon balm.

2. Detoxification & Body Therapies
Castor Oil Packs – Supports liver detox, reduces inflammation.
Hydration – Drink pure water, herbal teas, fresh juices, coconut water.
Sweating & Circulation – Sauna, steam, massage, rebounding, handstand yoga stool.
Lymphatic Support – Dry brushing, swimming, walking, yoga, breathwork.
Bath Therapy – Epsom salt baths, essential oil soaks.

3. Mind-Body Healing & Emotional Well-being
Stress Reduction – Meditation, breathwork, sound healing (528 Hz frequency).
Creative Expression – Poetry, painting, journaling.
Therapeutic Support – Counselling, energy healing, changing toxic environments (job, home, relationships).

4. Lifestyle & Energy Balance
Daily Movement – Yoga, rebounding, stretching, walking, swimming.
Sleep & Rest – Prioritize deep, restorative sleep and relaxation.
Eating & Drinking – Consume small, frequent meals to support digestion and energy levels.
Healing is a journey that requires commitment, patience, and a holistic approach. By nourishing the body, calming the mind, and creating a supportive environment, long-term wellness and balance can be achieved.

All about mental health…depression and bipolar [there are 586,396 papers on mental health, 667,391 on depression + 98,339 on bipolar + 170,894 on schizophrenia on pubmed.com]
Holistic Approach to Mental Health & Healing
Mental health challenges—bipolar disorder, depression, schizophrenia, anxiety, and OCD—are often the result of a complex interplay of trauma, stress, nutritional deficiencies, toxic overload, and physiological imbalances. Each individual's experience is unique, but healing is always possible with a multi-faceted approach that restores balance to the gut, nervous system, and adrenal glands.

1. Root Causes of Mental Health Struggles
Emotional & Environmental Factors – Trauma, stress, abuse, grief, spiritual crisis.
Physiological Imbalances – Chronic inflammation, infections, gut dysbiosis, oxidative stress (REDOX imbalance).
Hormonal & Adrenal Dysfunction – Elevated cortisol & adrenaline (fight-or-flight mode), high blood sugar fluctuations.
Nutritional Deficiencies – Depleted vitamins & minerals, poor absorption due to stress and gut damage.
Pharmaceutical Damage – Medications that impact liver function, gut microbiome, and metabolism.
Detox Pathways & Organ Congestion – Sluggish liver, congested lymphatic system, impaired digestion.

2. The Gut-Brain-Adrenal Connection

Serotonin (The "Happy" Hormone) – 95% is produced in the gut by the microbiome.

GABA (The "Calming" Hormone) – Primarily synthesized in the pancreas.

Stress & Gut Health – Chronic stress alters the microbiome, affecting neurotransmitter production and nutrient absorption.

Adrenal Fatigue & Nervous System Burnout – High cortisol and adrenaline levels keep the body in survival mode, disrupting digestion, metabolism, and sleep.

3. Steps to Healing the Mind & Body

A. Nutritional Support

Anti-Inflammatory Diet – Reduce sugar, processed foods, and high-carb meals; increase healthy fats.

Gut Healing Protocol – Restore microbiome balance with probiotics, digestive enzymes, and fermented foods.

Liver & Detox Support – Fresh juices, herbal teas, and liver-cleansing foods (e.g., lemon water, cruciferous vegetables, spirulina).

Nutrient-Dense Superfoods – Omega-3s, B vitamins, zinc, magnesium, amino acids, herbal adaptogens.

B. Stress Reduction & Nervous System Regulation

Rest & Sleep – Prioritize deep rest, relaxation, and circadian rhythm balance.

Breathwork & Meditation – Helps regulate cortisol, shift out of fight-or-flight mode.

Gentle Movement – Yoga, walking, swimming, rebounding to support lymphatic flow and adrenal health.

Sound Healing & Vibrational Therapy – 528 Hz music, grounding techniques, time in nature.

C. Emotional & Environmental Healing

Remove Toxic Triggers – Identify unhealthy relationships, toxic work environments, or emotional stressors.

D Therapeutic Outlets – Journaling, painting, poetry, creative expression.

Holistic Therapies – Castor oil packs, saunas, essential oil diffusion, energy healing practices.

Healing is a journey that requires commitment, self-care, and a supportive lifestyle. Small daily changes—starting with nutrition, relaxation, and mindful movement—can lead to profound transformation over time. Mental health is not just "in the mind"; it's deeply connected to the gut, nervous system, and overall body health.

The Path to True Healing

To heal, we must first understand the root causes of disease (*dis-ease*). At its core, illness stems from a combination of toxicity, stress, nutritional depletion, and physiological imbalances. Healing is not about masking symptoms but reversing damage at the cellular level through detoxification, nourishment, and lifestyle changes.

1. Root Causes of Disease

A. Oxidative Stress & REDOX Imbalance

An excess of free radicals and a lack of antioxidants leads to cellular damage, aging, and chronic illness.

Combated through antioxidant-rich foods, herbal detoxification, and mindful living.

B. Toxic Load & Environmental Pollutants

Heavy Metals – Mercury, lead, aluminium, cadmium (from industry, vaccines, amalgam fillings, food).

Chemical Exposure – Plastics, pesticides, household toxins, industrial pollutants.

Food Contaminants – Preservatives, additives, GMOs, artificial sweeteners, and processed oils.

C. Hidden Infections & Pathogens
Viruses & Bacteria – Epstein-Barr, Lyme, H. pylori, strep, etc.
Fungal Overgrowth – Candida, Mold toxicity.
Parasites & Protozoa – Often undetected but can drain nutrients and contribute to chronic illness.

D. Trauma, Stress & Emotional Health
Toxic Relationships & Emotional Wounds – Suppressed emotions manifest as illness.
Chronic Stress & Burnout – Triggers fight-or-flight mode, flooding the body with cortisol & adrenaline, leading to blood sugar imbalances, anxiety, and nervous system dysregulation.
Lack of Rest & Sleep – Inhibits healing, weakens immunity, and exacerbates inflammation.

E. Poor Diet & Nutritional Deficiencies
High-Sugar, High-Fat Diets – Lead to weight gain, sluggish organs, and systemic inflammation.
Processed & Artificial Foods – Disrupt gut microbiome, burden the liver, and contribute to disease.
Lymphatic & Liver Congestion – When detox pathways are blocked, the body cannot eliminate toxins effectively, leading to mucus buildup, inflammation, and disease proliferation.

2. Healing is a journey, not a Quick Fix

It is **not our fault** that we become sick. We live in a **toxic, high-stress world**, and illness is the natural consequence. **Food alone did not cause illness**, and reversing it requires a **multifaceted approach**:

✓ **Detox & Cleanse** – Remove accumulated toxins through herbal cleanses, juicing, and lymphatic support.

✓ **Nourish at a Cellular Level** – Prioritize organic, whole foods, healing herbs, and nutrient-dense superfoods.

✓ **Calm the Nervous System** – Reduce stress through breathwork, meditation, grounding, and restorative movement.

✓ **Support the Liver & Lymph** – Help the body eliminate waste through hydration, sweating (saunas, exercise), and detox baths.

✓ **Restore Gut Health** – Heal the microbiome with probiotics, fermented foods, and digestive support.

✓ **Prioritize Deep Rest & Recovery** – Healing requires **slow, intentional** living. Sleep, relaxation, and joy are vital.

Healing is the **undoing of years of damage**—but the **body knows how to heal** when given the right tools. Start small, be consistent, and build healing habits **step by step**. The knowledge to restore health **is here, and it is within your power.** 🌿✨

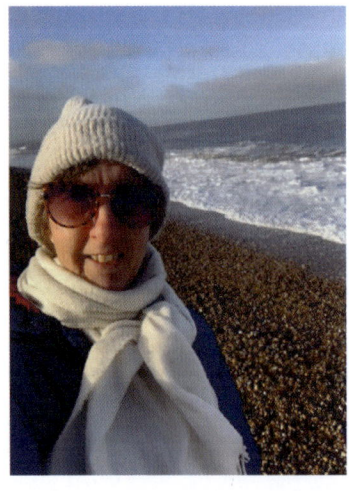

Detox + Cleanse
1 Lemon water or ginger water
2 Celery juice or cucumber + apple
3 Heavy metal detox smoothie
1 banana + juice 1 orange +
Detox powder = Atlantic dulce +
Spirulina + barley grass juice powder
½ cup of coriander + cup of blueberries
4 avocado + asparagus salad etc
5 fresh herbs + spices + roots
6 ginger + turmeric + garlic
7 real honey + real maple syrup
8 veg tray bakes + hot pots
9 olive oil + coconut oil sparingly
10 dark chocolate 85% + medjool dates
11 home-made apple + pear sauce
12 soups + salads + smoothies + juicing

JUICING
celery [build slowly up to a pint a day]
1 cucumber + 2 apples or 2 pears + mint
2 oranges + 7 carrots + ginger + turmeric
1 cucumber + 1 head celery + 1 lemon
4 apples + [parsley or coriander]
1 courgette + 2 apples + cucumber
EXTRAS....spinach + kale + broccoli
fennel + lettuce + cabbage + sprouts
coconut water + herbals teas
hibiscus + camomile + aloe vera water
basil & other fresh herbs & roots etc
increasing hydration increases the
flow, so cleanses the cells

SMOOTHIES
heavy metal detox smoothies
frozen red berries
gluten free oats + chia seeds
pumpkin seeds + flax seeds
soaked almonds + other nuts
spices + roots + ashwagandha
goji berries + coconut water
avocado + coconut + fruits
coconut milk + spinach
black strap molasses
kale + spices + roots
leafy greens
sea weeds + dulce etc

PATHOGENS + TOXICITIES
viruses + bacteria + fungi
yeasts + candida + Mold
parasites + heavy metals
chemicals + farming + foods
water + air + personal products
furniture + clothes + perfume
candles + pharmaceuticals
avoid as much as you can
house hold sprays + cleaners
cooking in tin foil + non-stick pans
lead in paint + petrol + pipes etc
mercury in fish etc
chemicals in caffeine-free coffee

WEAN OFF
eggs + dairy + sugar
sweeteners + grains
alcohol + coffee
black tea + fizzy drinks
pork + soy + vinegar
fermented foods
milk chocolate
pastry + bread
rice + pasta
man-made foods
squash
muesli + granola
food in tins + jars

All about autism and ADHD [the are 81,520 on autism + 52,815 on ADHD on pubmed.com]

Understanding and Healing Autism, ADHD, and Epilepsy

Neurodevelopmental conditions such as Autism, ADHD, and Epilepsy are not isolated disorders but complex conditions with multiple root causes. These conditions often stem from a combination of toxicity, infections, gut dysfunction, immune dysregulation, and nutritional deficiencies. While every individual is unique, many of the underlying triggers overlap across these conditions, making holistic healing possible.

1. Autism: A Multifactorial Condition

Autism Spectrum Disorder (ASD) is influenced by a variety of biological and environmental factors that disrupt neurodevelopment. While genetics play a small role, epigenetics (environmental influences on gene expression) are key drivers.

A. Underlying Causes & Contributing Factors

Bacterial Biofilms & Pathogens – Chronic infections (Lyme, strep, mycoplasma, Epstein-Barr) disrupt neurodevelopment and contribute to gut-brain inflammation.

Toxicity Overload – Heavy metals (aluminium, mercury), plastics, pesticides, and environmental chemicals impair detoxification and neurological function.

Allergies & Sensitivities – Many children with autism react to gluten, dairy, artificial additives, household toxins, and Mold, worsening symptoms.

Maternal Health & Prenatal Exposure – The mother's toxic load, stress levels, gut health, and nutrient status during pregnancy directly affect foetal brain development.

Inflammation & Immune Dysfunction – Many children with autism have mast cell activation syndrome (MCAS), causing skin issues, gut problems, and sensory processing difficulties.

B. Key Healing Strategies

Gut Healing & Microbiome Support – Reduce inflammation with probiotic-rich foods, fermented foods, and gut-repairing nutrients (glutamine, bone broth, colostrum).

Anti-Inflammatory Nutrition – Eliminate processed foods, artificial additives, gluten, dairy, and soy while increasing omega-3s, fresh fruits, and vegetables.

Reduce Toxic Load – Swap chemical-laden household cleaners, personal care products, and plastics for natural alternatives.

Address Infections & Detox Pathways – Natural antimicrobials (oregano oil, black seed oil, colloidal silver) help clear pathogens, while liver support (milk thistle, dandelion) aids detoxification.

Nervous System Regulation – Sound therapy, sensory integration, and movement-based therapies improve brain function and emotional regulation.

2. ADHD: Overlapping Causes with Autism

Attention Deficit Hyperactivity Disorder (ADHD) shares many root causes with autism, particularly dopamine dysregulation and heightened nervous system activity.

A. Contributing Factors

Oxidative Stress & Neuroinflammation – Chronic inflammation disrupts focus, impulse control, and executive function.

Gut Dysfunction & Nutrient Deficiencies – Low B vitamins, magnesium, omega-3s, zinc, and iron impact neurotransmitter production and regulation.

Toxic Exposures in Utero & Childhood – Heavy metals, artificial dyes, pesticides, and EMF exposure can exacerbate hyperactivity and attention issues.

Dopamine & Serotonin Imbalances – Dopamine (produced in the adrenals & hypothalamus) and serotonin (made 95% in the gut) influence mood, attention, and behaviour.

B. Healing Strategies

Dopamine-Supportive Foods – Protein-rich foods, tyrosine-containing foods (bananas, almonds), and omega-3s (wild salmon, flaxseeds) boost dopamine levels.

Eliminate Hyperactivity Triggers – Remove processed foods, synthetic dyes, MSG, and artificial sweeteners to stabilize mood and focus.

Support Detox Pathways – Sauna therapy, Epsom salt baths, and lymphatic movement (rebounding, dry brushing) aid in toxin removal.

Regulate the Nervous System – Breathwork, meditation, and nature exposure help calm an overactive stress response and improve emotional regulation.

3. Epilepsy: The Role of Inflammation & Electrical Dysfunction

Epilepsy is often linked to brain inflammation, gut permeability, immune dysfunction, and heavy **metal toxicity.**

A. Root Causes & Contributing Factors

Neuroinflammation & Mast Cell Activation – Excessive electrical activity in the brain can be triggered by chronic inflammation and immune dysfunction.

Parasites & Infections – Chronic viral and bacterial infections can contribute to seizures by disrupting neuronal signalling.

Heavy Metal Toxicity – Mercury, lead, and aluminium interfere with the brain's electrical stability.

Nutritional Deficiencies – Low B12, magnesium, and omega-3s are common in those with epilepsy and can trigger neurological instability.

Antibiotic Overuse in Childhood – Weakens gut integrity, contributes to immune dysfunction, and affects neurotransmitter balance.

B. Healing Strategies

Anti-Inflammatory Diet – A ketogenic-style diet rich in healthy fats (avocados, coconut oil, grass-fed butter) can stabilize brain electrical activity and reduce seizures.

Gut Healing & Immune Support – Probiotics, colostrum, and fermented foods restore gut barrier integrity and strengthen the immune system.

Magnesium & B12 Supplementation – Supports neuronal function and reduces seizure frequency.

Detoxification & Heavy Metal Removal – Chlorella, cilantro, and binders like zeolite help eliminate neurotoxic metals and support detox pathways.

4. Healing Is a Journey, Not an Overnight Fix

Children with autism, ADHD, and epilepsy often experience sensory sensitivities, food aversions, and resistance to change. Healing requires patience, consistency, and gradual changes in daily habits.

Practical Steps for Parents & Caregivers

Start Small – Introduce new foods through smoothies and juices to increase nutrient intake without overwhelming the child.

Reduce Triggers – Swap chemical cleaners, personal care products, and food additives for natural alternatives to minimize toxic exposure.

Educate & Empower – Explain changes to the child in a way they can understand, making healing a collaborative process.

Be Patient & Flexible – Every child is different; progress happens step by step.

5. The Gut-Brain Connection: Key to Healing

Neurotransmitters are not just made in the brain—they are deeply influenced by gut health, adrenal function, and immune regulation.

Serotonin (95%) is produced in the gut microbiome.

Dopamine is synthesized in the adrenals and hypothalamus.

GABA, a calming neurotransmitter, is also made in the gut microbiome.

With the right diet, detoxification, and nervous system support, healing is always possible. 🌿✨

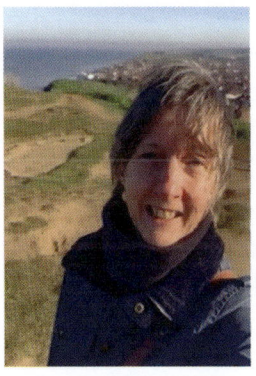

Detox + Cleanse
1 Lemon water or ginger water
2 Celery juice or cucumber + apple
3 Heavy metal detox smoothie
1 banana + juice 1 orange +
Detox powder = Atlantic dulce +
Spirulina + barley grass juice powder
½ cup of coriander + cup of blueberries
4 avocado + asparagus salad etc
5 fresh herbs + spices + roots
6 ginger + turmeric + garlic
7 real honey + real maple syrup
8 veg tray bakes + hot pots
9 olive oil + coconut oil sparingly
10 dark chocolate 85% + medjool dates
11 home-made apple + pear sauce
12 soups + salads + smoothies + juicing

JUICING
celery [build slowly up to a pint a day]
1 cucumber + 2 apples or 2 pears + mint
2 oranges + 7 carrots + ginger + turmeric
1 cucumber + 1 head celery + 1 lemon
4 apples + [parsley or coriander]
1 courgette + 2 apples + cucumber
EXTRAS....spinach + kale + broccoli
fennel + lettuce + cabbage + sprouts
coconut water + herbals teas
hibiscus + camomile + aloe vera water
basil & other fresh herbs & roots etc
increasing hydration increases the
flow, so cleanses the cells

SMOOTHIES	PATHOGENS + TOXICITIES	WEAN OFF
heavy metal detox smoothies	viruses + bacteria + fungi	eggs + dairy + sugar
frozen red berries	yeasts + candida + Mold	sweeteners + grains
gluten free oats + chia seeds	parasites + heavy metals	alcohol + coffee
pumpkin seeds + flax seeds	chemicals + farming + foods	black tea + fizzy drinks
soaked almonds + other nuts	water + air + personal products	pork + soy + vinegar
spices + roots + ashwagandha	furniture + clothes + perfume	fermented foods
goji berries + coconut water	candles + pharmaceuticals	milk chocolate
avocado + coconut + fruits	avoid as much as you can	pastry + bread
coconut milk + spinach	house hold sprays + cleaners	rice + pasta
black strap molasses	cooking in tin foil + non-stick pans	man-made foods
kale + spices + roots	lead in paint + petrol + pipes etc	squash
leafy greens	mercury in fish etc	muesli + granola
sea weeds + dulce etc	chemicals in caffeine-free coffee	food in tins + jars

Supporting Children with Autism, ADHD, and Epilepsy Through Nutrition and Lifestyle
Working daily on incorporating juices, smoothies, and healing recipes into a child's diet can bring significant benefits—helping to stabilize moods, improve sleep, and restore balance to the gut microbiome. These foundational changes are key to making progress with these complex conditions.
Engaging children in food preparation through messy play and fun cooking activities can make the process more enjoyable and effective than lengthy discussions. Encouraging creativity in the kitchen builds positive associations with new foods while reducing resistance to dietary changes. Beyond nutrition, movement and relaxation play an essential role in calming an overstimulated nervous system. Activities such as swimming, nature walks, seaside visits, and sensory play can provide much-needed grounding and emotional regulation. A quiet, low-stimulation environment— free from excessive screen time, loud noises, and over-talking—can help children feel more at ease. Hydration and balanced blood sugar levels are also critical. Encouraging children to eat small, frequent meals prevents energy crashes and mood swings that can lead to irritability and overeating.

Creating a home environment free from synthetic chemicals, artificial fragrances, and toxic cleaning sprays is equally important, as many children with these conditions are highly sensitive to environmental toxins. Opting for natural materials such as cotton bedding and clothing over synthetic fabrics can further reduce irritants.

Supplementing with a high-quality, buffered vitamin C powder can support the body's ability to combat oxidative stress. Easily added to a drink, this simple daily step provides a powerful antioxidant boost that aids in reducing inflammation and supporting immune function.

By combining these dietary and lifestyle shifts with patience and consistency, caregivers can help children feel more balanced, supported, and nourished laying the foundation for long-term healing and well-being.

AUTISM
Mitochondrial dysfunction =omega 3 fatty acids, multi vitamins, minerals & nutritional supplements.
Chronic neuroinflammation/ increased cytokines = anti-inflammatory diet & supplements.
Oxidative stress/redox imbalance = antioxidant foods & supplements.
Hormonal imbalances = healing the gut dysbiosis.
Glutamate/GABAergic imbalance = healing the gut dysbiosis.
Dysregulation of monoaminergic neurotransmission = healing the gut dysbiosis.
Immune dysregulation = healing the gut dysregulation.
Environmental toxins & stressors = chelating agents, anti-stress practices & heavy metal detox smoothie, zeolites.

ADHD.
Evidence of inflammation.
Allergic diseases.
Maternal immune activation during pregnancy.
Immune mediated disorders.
Inflammatory biochemical markers in blood.
Co aggregation of ADHD, auto immune diseases among relatives.
Auto immune diseases.
Oxidative stress/redox imbalance.
Inflammatory biochemical markers in cerebrospinal fluid.

All about Alzheimer's, dementia and Parkinson's [there are 241,893 papers on Alzheimer's + 295,012 on dementia + 184,526 on Parkinson's at pubmed.com]

Brain Health and Neurodegenerative Conditions

Conditions such as dementia, Alzheimer's, ALS, motor neuron disease, and Parkinson's often stem from a combination of factors, including toxicities, heavy metals, free radical oxidative stress (REDOX imbalance), depleted nutrition, inflammation, gut dysbiosis, pharmaceutical damage, infections, pathogens, and blood sugar dysregulation.

We live in an increasingly toxic world, and multiple environmental and lifestyle factors contribute to brain disease. Research available on **PubMed.com** highlights many of these root causes. While every individual is unique, addressing these underlying issues can significantly improve brain health and slow or even reverse cognitive decline.

Healing the Brain Through the Gut

Since many neurotransmitters are produced in the gut, restoring gut health is a crucial step in supporting brain function. Altering the microbiome with fresh herbs, juicing, and the **heavy metal detox smoothie** can help calm the nervous system, provide essential nutrients for the brain, and support the body's natural detoxification processes.

A **natural, anti-inflammatory diet** that avoids processed foods, high-fat meals, and dehydrating drinks is vital for protecting cognitive function. Many older adults struggle to properly digest grains and heavy, fat-laden meals, which can contribute to sluggish metabolism and increased toxicity. Instead, focusing on **juicing, fresh herbs, fruits, smoothies, and soups** can aid digestion, enhance hydration, and support detoxification.

Antioxidant Support and Hydration
Oxidative stress plays a significant role in neurodegenerative conditions, making it essential to **rebalance antioxidants** in the body. A diet rich in alkaline, whole foods—such as **fruits, vegetables, fresh greens, and salads**—can help combat inflammation and protect brain cells from damage. Super-hydration through juicing is one of the easiest ways to deliver essential nutrients directly to the cells, bypassing the strain of digestion.

Fresh herbs also play a powerful role in cleansing the body of pathogens, parasites, and toxic substances, all of which contribute to cognitive decline. By improving gut health and reducing inflammation, the brain can regain its ability to function optimally.

With the right approach—**hydration, detoxification, and nutrient-dense foods**—it is possible to restore and maintain brain health, even in later years.

The Daily Cleansing choices + Healing Protocol
Morning Hydration Options
Lemon or Ginger Water + Thyme, or any real herbal tea of your choice. You can add real honey or maple syrup for a touch of sweetness.

Homemade Apple + Pear Sauce
Add spices like cinnamon, cloves, nutmeg, or fresh ginger for extra flavour and warmth.

Celery Juice
Start with ½ cup, and gradually build up to a full pint per day over 2 weeks.

Juicing Combo
5 Carrots
2 Oranges
1 tsp of real turmeric
1-inch piece of fresh ginger

Heavy Metal Detox Smoothie
1 cup blueberries
1 or 2 bananas
Juice of 1 or 2 oranges
½ cup coriander
1 tsp spirulina
1 tsp Atlantic dulce
1 tsp barley grass juice powder

Salads & Veggies
Salad with avocado, leafy greens, asparagus, garlic, and any salad of your choice.
Homemade dressing with olive oil and vinegar.
Roasted vegetable soup (e.g., butternut squash, sweet potatoes).

Snacks & Treats
Medjool Dates + Coconut Water

Lynn's Homemade Hot Chocolate:
1 Medjool date
1 tsp gluten-free oats
1 square dark chocolate (85%)
Water
Cinnamon
Maple syrup or honey

Lynn's Homemade Flapjacks:
GF oats
Maple syrup or honey
Medjool dates
Dark chocolate

Lynn's Homemade Fruit Crumble: Use fresh or frozen fruits, a GF oat topping, and a touch of maple syrup for sweetness.

Hearty Meals
Hot Pots & Tray Bakes: Rich, Savory meals packed with root vegetables and your choice of protein.
Soups: Wholesome, comforting varieties like butternut squash and sweet potato.
Juicing & Smoothies: Regular additions to your daily routine to boost health with fresh fruits and veggies.

Fats & Oils
Use coconut oil and olive oil for cooking or as dressings to add healthy fats to your meals.

Spices & Herbs
Fresh ginger, garlic, turmeric, and other fresh herbs and spices to enhance flavour and health benefits.

Detox + Cleanse
1 Lemon water or ginger water
2 Celery juice or cucumber + apple
3 Heavy metal detox smoothie
1 banana + juice 1 orange +
Detox powder = Atlantic dulce +
Spirulina + barley grass juice powder
½ cup of coriander + cup of blueberries
4 avocado + asparagus salad etc
5 fresh herbs + spices + roots
6 ginger + turmeric + garlic
7 real honey + real maple syrup
8 veg tray bakes + hot pots
9 olive oil + coconut oil sparingly
10 dark chocolate 85% + medjool dates
11 home-made apple + pear sauce
12 soups + salads + smoothies + juicing

JUICING
celery [build slowly up to a pint a day]
1 cucumber + 2 apples or 2 pears + mint
2 oranges + 7 carrots + ginger + turmeric
1 cucumber + 1 head celery + 1 lemon
4 apples + [parsley or coriander]
1 courgette + 2 apples + cucumber
EXTRAS....spinach + kale + broccoli
fennel + lettuce + cabbage + sprouts
coconut water + herbals teas
hibiscus + camomile + aloe vera water
basil & other fresh herbs & roots etc
increasing hydration increases the
flow, so cleanses the cells

SMOOTHIES	PATHOGENS + TOXICITIES	WEAN OFF
heavy metal detox smoothies	viruses + bacteria + fungi	eggs + dairy + sugar
frozen red berries	yeasts + candida + Mold	sweeteners + grains
gluten free oats + chia seeds	parasites + heavy metals	alcohol + coffee
pumpkin seeds + flax seeds	chemicals + farming + foods	black tea + fizzy drinks
soaked almonds + other nuts	water + air + personal products	pork + soy + vinegar
spices + roots + ashwagandha	furniture + clothes + perfume	fermented foods
goji berries + coconut water	candles + pharmaceuticals	milk chocolate
avocado + coconut + fruits	avoid as much as you can	pastry + bread
coconut milk + spinach	house hold sprays + cleaners	rice + pasta
black strap molasses	cooking in tin foil + non-stick pans	man-made foods
kale + spices + roots	lead in paint + petrol + pipes etc	squash
leafy greens	mercury in fish etc	muesli + granola
sea weeds + dulce etc	chemicals in caffeine-free coffee	food in tins + jars

All about diabetes and the gall bladder

Diabetes type two is insulin resistance, caused by a high carbohydrate diet, a stagnant, congested liver, with maybe pathogens and toxicities its harbouring. can be a weight issues, but not always, a low carbohydrate diet is need. Type one diabetes is an infection that has destroyed the pancreas, like an auto immune dis ease, to use less insulin and avoid another auto immune dis ease on top, blood sugars need to be kept low, so a low carbohydrate diet is needed. Type two is reversible, but type one is better managed but not reversible. Gall bladder is poor digestion and also a stagnant, sluggish pathogen filled liver, can be parasites and bacteria and pathogens. A low fat, low carbohydrate diet is needed.

0% TOP	10%.	20%.	50%. TOP	75%.	90%.	100%
Fish.	Overground veg.	Underground veg.	2 slices Bread		Pastry.	Sugar
Meat.	Cauliflower.	Potatoes	Beans	Pizza.	Milk chocolate	
Eggs.	Broccoli.	Sweet potatoes.	Pasta	Cereals	Meringues	
Mushrooms	sprouts.	Bananas.	Rice	Honey.	Cereals	
Seafood.	Avocados	Grapes	1/2 cup oats		Maple syrup	
Dairy (?).	Green beans	Mangoes	Flax seed 30g	Dates		
Cold meats.	Melons	Lentils	Chia 40g			
Coconut oil	Blueberries	Cashews	Wraps			
Olive oil	Strawberries	Almonds				
Cucumber.	Raspberries					
Courgette	Butternut squash					
Lettuce.	Carrots					
Bok Choi.	Oranges					
Spinach.	Tangerines					
Cabbage						
Asparagus						
Peppers						
Kale/spinach						
Tomatoes						
Radishes						

As you can see, these are rough estimates of the carbohydrate values in various foods. Carbohydrates represent the glucose/sugar content of foods, and it's the high-carb ones that can contribute to insulin resistance and a high-fat diet. When planning meals, swapping high-carb foods for low-carb alternatives is key to lowering blood sugar levels over time and can help in reversing type 2 diabetes.

It's also important to gradually reduce or eliminate foods like dairy, bacon, sausages, and eggs from your diet. Sugar is often hidden in many products, such as ice cream, pasta sauces, and processed foods, so it's crucial to reduce your intake of these gradually. A keto diet can be particularly beneficial for managing diabetes, and the same principle applies to gallbladder issues.

To help with both weight and blood sugar management, it's best to wean off grains like bread, pasta, rice, and oats. Instead, focus on meals based around vegetables like sweet potatoes, cauliflower, broccoli, and carrots. Overground vegetables are generally lower in carbs, but root vegetables like butternut squash are also acceptable.

During the process of cutting out grains, you may find that you need to eat more to stay satisfied. Fill up on vegetables, mushrooms, and meats (if you eat them). Keep in mind that dairy, pork, and fatty meats like mince are high in fat, so it's best to reduce these and opt for healthier choices. Fruit is okay in moderation, especially red berries, which are rich in antioxidants and beneficial for diabetes management. A diet focused on healthy fruits and vegetables is crucial for managing metabolic illnesses.

The recipes in this book are suitable for those with diabetes. Additionally, it's advisable to wean off coffee, alcohol, and fizzy drinks—especially those labelled as "sugar-free." These often contain artificial sweeteners, which can hinder liver healing and overall health.

HEALING + SUPPLEMENTS: Holistic Healing Practices

Nutrition & Detoxification: Focus on a nutrient-dense, anti-inflammatory diet rich in fresh vegetables, fruits, and herbs.

Yoga & Breathwork: Incorporate yoga, breathwork, and sound healing (528 Hz) to promote relaxation and balance.

Essential Oils: Use a diffuser with essential oils to support emotional and physical healing.

Hydrotherapy: Include practices like baths, sauna, steam, and swimming to support detoxification and relaxation.

Massage & Rebounding: Massage therapy and rebounding (mini trampoline exercises) can enhance circulation and detox.

Exercise: Regular physical activity such as walking and yoga (using a handstand yoga stool for variation) promotes overall wellness.

Mental and Emotional Health

Counselling & Journaling: Engage in therapy or counselling, and reflect through journaling to support mental health.

Creativity: Activities like poetry and painting can help express and release emotions.

Life Changes: Consider positive life changes, such as a new job, moving home, or improving relationships, for overall happiness and stress reduction.

Spices, Herbs & Supplements

Roots & Fresh Herbs: Include turmeric, ginger, garlic, and fresh herbs like lemon balm and oregano in your diet.

Nutrient Boosters: Support your body with supplements like Vitamin C, D, B12, zinc, spirulina, barley grass juice powder, and Atlantic dulce.

Immune Support: Herbs like echinacea, elderberry, goldenseal, and black walnut hulls help bolster immunity.

Adaptogens & Stress Support: Use ashwagandha, ginseng, and CBD oil for stress resilience.

Gut Health: Probiotics, prebiotics, and digestive enzymes aid digestion and gut health.

Liver Support: Milk thistle and NAC (N-acetyl cysteine) support detoxification.

Antioxidants: Astaxanthin, rosehip, and chaga mushrooms provide powerful antioxidant benefits.

Essential Fatty Acids & Natural Remedies
Omega-3 Oils: Support brain and heart health with omega-3 fatty acids.
Herbal Teas: Drink calming and healing herbal teas such as hibiscus, chamomile, and lemon balm.
Natural Sweeteners: Use real honey and maple syrup in moderation for natural sweetness.
Additional Healing Support: Black seed oil, liquorice, L-lysine, GABA, CoQ10, and glutathione can offer various health benefits.
Self-Care & Wellness Practices
Castor Oil Packs: Use castor oil packs to promote lymphatic drainage and liver detox.
Hydration & Rest: Maintain adequate hydration, rest, relaxation, and sleep for overall wellness.
Eating & Drinking Habits: Eat and drink little and often to maintain steady energy levels and metabolic function.

All about high blood pressure and high cholesterol [there are 766,109 papers on high blood pressure + 166,187 on high cholesterol on pubmed.com]

High Blood Pressure:
High blood pressure is often a result of thick, dehydrated blood. When the blood becomes thick, the liver becomes overburdened, and blood is drawn from the liver to the heart. As the liver struggles to function effectively, the heart has to work harder, which increases blood pressure. The root cause of high blood pressure often lies within the liver (and kidneys), which can be compromised by various factors such as pathogens, a high-fat diet, excessive alcohol, coffee, fizzy drinks, salt, vinegar, and weight issues related to a high-carbohydrate, sugar, and grain-based diet.
The liver becomes sluggish and stagnant due to toxicities, pathogens, and an improper diet. A diet rich in grains, dairy, and sugar contributes to a congested and sluggish liver that has difficulty processing and detoxifying efficiently.
To Lower Blood Pressure and Heal:
To address high blood pressure, we must focus on addressing weight issues and improving liver function. A low-carbohydrate, low-sugar, and low-grain diet is essential, which includes gradually eliminating foods like grains, sugar, unhealthy fats (e.g., deep-fried foods), dairy, pork, and eggs.
Key dietary changes to support liver health and reduce blood pressure:
Hydration: Focus on proper hydration with water, fresh juices, and herbal teas sweetened with real honey or maple syrup.
Weaning Off Processed Foods: Gradually eliminate dairy, pasta, pizza, bread, and rice. Instead, choose nutrient-dense root vegetables like butternut squash, sweet potatoes, carrots, and parsnips.
Healthy Fats: Swap vegetable and seed oils for healthier options like olive oil and coconut oil, used sparingly.
Weight Management: Achieving and maintaining a healthy weight is crucial for supporting liver function and lowering blood pressure.

High Cholesterol:
High cholesterol is often an indication of a liver struggling to process a high-fat diet or dealing with pathogens like bacteria, yeasts, viruses, fungi, and parasites. Additionally, dehydration caused by poor drink choices—such as coffee, black tea, alcohol, and fizzy drinks—can exacerbate the problem.

Cholesterol Issues and Gall Bladder Health:
Cholesterol imbalances can lead to problems with the gall bladder, including the formation of gallstones and associated pain. To support liver health and aid in the healing process, consider supplements like milk thistle, known for its liver-protective properties.

Dietary Changes for Healing:
Eliminating bad fats, such as pork, trans fats, and deep-fried foods, is essential. Gradually wean these out of your diet to allow your body to transition into a healthier state.

Supportive Nutrition:
Incorporating juicing and smoothies can help boost blood flow and provide much-needed nutrients to a fatty, congested liver. These practices support the detoxification process and can assist in restoring liver function over time.

Patience in the Healing Process:
It's important to understand that it takes time for high cholesterol and high blood pressure to develop, and similarly, it will take time to see the healing results. Reversing metabolic health issues, such as cholesterol imbalances, requires addressing multiple factors: stress, diet, pathogens, toxicities, and weight issues. By following a consistent, healthy protocol, these issues are reversible, but it will take time.

Regular Health Monitoring:
As you make these changes, always remember to have regular check-ups with your healthcare provider to track your progress and adjust as needed.

HEALING + SUPPLEMENTS

Holistic Healing Approach:
Achieving overall health and wellness requires a multifaceted approach that integrates nutrition, detoxification, and self-care practices. By nourishing the body and mind, we create a balanced environment for healing and thriving.

Physical Practices:
Yoga (including handstand stool yoga)
Breathwork
Exercise (walking, swimming, rebounding)
Sauna & Steam
Massage
Baths
Castor Oil Packs
Emotional & Mental Well-Being:
Counselling
Journaling
Poetry
Painting
Stress Management (changing jobs, home, or relationships)

Nutritional Support:
Hydration (water, herbal teas with honey or maple syrup)
Eating Little & Often
Juicing & Smoothies (incorporating nutrient-dense vegetables, fruits, and herbs)
Salads & Soups
Spices & Fresh Herbs (turmeric, ginger, garlic, etc.)
Nutrient-Rich Foods:
Vegetables
Vitamin C & D
B12
Zinc
Spirulina & Barley Grass Juice Powder
Chaga Mushrooms
Atlantic Dulce & Kelp
Healing Supplements:
Milk Thistle (for liver health)
Omega-3 Oils
L-lysine, GABA, Glutathione, CoQ10
Ashwagandha & CBD Oil (for stress support)
NAC (N-acetyl cysteine)
Pro & Prebiotics
Digestive Enzymes
Echinacea, Elderberry, Cat's Claw
Black Seed Oil, Liquorice, Black Walnut Hulls
Hibiscus, Camomile, Rose Hip (herbal teas)
Astaxanthin
Turmeric, Ginger, Cinnamon (for inflammation and digestion)
Detoxification Support:
Essential Oils (via diffuser)
Sound Healing (528 Hz frequency)
Herbal Remedies (Goldenseal, Oregano Oil)
Lifestyle Practices:
Rest & Relaxation (quality sleep)
Time Outdoors (sunlight for vitamin D, fresh air for healing)
By combining these practices and making them a part of your daily routine, you support your body's natural healing process, balance stress, and nurture mental, emotional, and physical well-being.

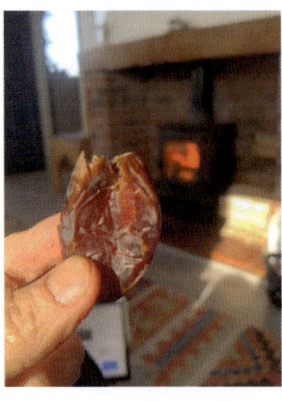

Detox + Cleanse
1 Lemon water or ginger water
2 Celery juice or cucumber + apple
3 Heavy metal detox smoothie
1 banana + juice 1 orange +
Detox powder = Atlantic dulce +
Spirulina + barley grass juice powder
½ cup of coriander + cup of blueberries
4 avocado + asparagus salad etc
5 fresh herbs + spices + roots
6 ginger + turmeric + garlic
7 real honey + real maple syrup
8 veg tray bakes + hot pots
9 olive oil + coconut oil sparingly
10 dark chocolate 85% + medjool dates
11 home-made apple + pear sauce
12 soups + salads + smoothies + juicing

JUICING
celery [build slowly up to a pint a day]
1 cucumber + 2 apples or 2 pears + mint
2 oranges + 7 carrots + ginger + turmeric
1 cucumber + 1 head celery + 1 lemon
4 apples + [parsley or coriander]
1 courgette + 2 apples + cucumber
EXTRAS....spinach + kale + broccoli
fennel + lettuce + cabbage + sprouts
coconut water + herbals teas
hibiscus + camomile + aloe vera water
basil & other fresh herbs & roots etc
increasing hydration increases the
flow, so cleanses the cells

SMOOTHIES	**PATHOGENS + TOXICITIES**	**WEAN OFF**
heavy metal detox smoothies	viruses + bacteria + fungi	eggs + dairy + sugar
frozen red berries	yeasts + candida + Mold	sweeteners + grains
gluten free oats + chia seeds	parasites + heavy metals	alcohol + coffee
pumpkin seeds + flax seeds	chemicals + farming + foods	black tea + fizzy drinks
soaked almonds + other nuts	water + air + personal products	pork + soy + vinegar
spices + roots + ashwagandha	furniture + clothes + perfume	fermented foods
goji berries + coconut water	candles + pharmaceuticals	milk chocolate
avocado + coconut + fruits	avoid as much as you can	pastry + bread
coconut milk + spinach	house hold sprays + cleaners	rice + pasta
black strap molasses	cooking in tin foil + non-stick pans	man-made foods
kale + spices + roots	lead in paint + petrol + pipes etc	squash
leafy greens	mercury in fish etc	muesli + granola
sea weeds + dulce etc	chemicals in caffeine-free coffee	food in tins + jars

When we break it down, the root causes of many health problems become clear. A liver in need of extra care and gentle cleansing is often at the core of chronic conditions. While each person's healing journey is unique, the underlying causes are often similar, and they can be addressed. With consistent effort, we can rise in health by practicing daily healing.

Choosing better foods and drinks that support our bodies is essential, especially in today's world, where we are exposed to unhealthy chemicals and toxins more than ever before. Unfortunately, issues like high blood pressure and cholesterol are now affecting people at younger ages, but these problems are not genetic. We can take control by making better choices.

PubMed.com is a great resource for peer-reviewed scientific research, offering valuable insights into which foods, supplements, and protocols can help us reverse chronic conditions and find remission. In this book, I'll outline protocols and provide simple, delicious recipes for all tastes—recipes that are easy to prepare, pack up, and support healing. Preparation is key in any healing journey. The small changes we make each day shape our long-term health outcomes, and it's those repeated changes that become our new habits, helping our bodies and minds thrive.

Our immune systems are facing more threats today than ever before. The blood and lymphatic systems need constant care and attention to keep them clean and functioning properly. In colder climates, it's especially important to maintain a high-quality vitamin D level in winter, as it helps protect us from infections like the flu and even COVID.

The holiday season—filled with overindulgence in unhealthy foods and drinks—can lead to congestion, mucus buildup, and the proliferation of pathogens in our bodies. Our body naturally tries to purge toxins through symptoms like fever, a runny nose, or digestive discomfort. During this time, it's essential to support the body with healing practices like drinking fresh herbal teas, boosting vitamin C, and incorporating immune-supportive ingredients like echinacea, garlic, ginger, and turmeric into our meals and soups.

By being mindful of what we eat and drink, supporting our liver, and committing to small, consistent changes, we can help our bodies detoxify and thrive in the face of modern challenges.

All about menopause, endometriosis, fibroids and PCOS [there are 99,261 papers on menopause + 36,559 on endometriosis + 31,119 on fibroids + 17,564 on PCOS on pubmed.com]

Menopause often stems from a combination of weak adrenals, an underactive thyroid, a stagnant liver, poor metabolic health, poor diet, and insulin resistance. These factors can make the transition more difficult and contribute to symptoms. Fibroids, on the other hand, can result from pathogens, viruses, chemicals, bacteria, and thyroid imbalances. Endometriosis is similarly influenced by pathogens, viruses, bacteria, chemicals, and stress. PCOS is linked to toxicities, pathogens, and dysregulated metabolism. PMS can be exacerbated by hormone-disrupting foods, drinks, pathogens, and toxicities.

Common symptoms like mood swings, brain fog, and hot flashes are often the result of blood sugar dysregulation, insulin resistance, pathogens, toxicities, a sluggish liver, and dehydration.

It's easy to blame the perimenopause or menopause for these symptoms, as it's a convenient scapegoat. The natural expectation is that the adrenals will take over after the ovaries slow down. However, many women experience high cortisol due to stress, which can overwhelm the adrenals and other organs like the liver and pancreas. Over the years, the accumulation of other health issues may intensify during menopause, leading to a host of additional challenges.

We live in an increasingly toxic world, and women are particularly sensitive to environmental toxins like those found in cleaning products, personal care products, and chemicals in food. Medications, including birth control, can also have long-term side effects that contribute to health issues.

The best way to support a struggling body is by embracing a more ancestral diet, similar to what our great-grandmothers would have eaten. This includes focusing on fresh herbs, fruits, vegetables, soups, and juicing to help cleanse the body and regulate hormones. Unfortunately, many foods we're told are healthy—like dairy, eggs, grains, and refined sugars—can actually impede healing by congesting the body and driving insulin resistance. Instead, opt for natural sweeteners like real honey or maple syrup, which are gentler on the body.

By addressing these root causes and following a thoughtful detox plan, you can begin to regulate your body and restore balance, helping to ease the struggles that come with menopause and beyond.

Detox + Cleanse
1 Lemon water or ginger water
2 Celery juice or cucumber + apple
3 Heavy metal detox smoothie
1 banana + juice 1 orange +
Detox powder = Atlantic dulce +
Spirulina + barley grass juice powder
½ cup of coriander + cup of blueberries
4 avocado + asparagus salad etc
5 fresh herbs + spices + roots
6 ginger + turmeric + garlic
7 real honey + real maple syrup
8 veg tray bakes + hot pots
9 olive oil + coconut oil sparingly
10 dark chocolate 85% + medjool dates
11 home-made apple + pear sauce
12 soups + salads + smoothies + juicing

JUICING
celery [build slowly up to a pint a day]
1 cucumber + 2 apples or 2 pears + mint
2 oranges + 7 carrots + ginger + turmeric
1 cucumber + 1 head celery + 1 lemon
4 apples + [parsley or coriander]
1 courgette + 2 apples + cucumber
EXTRAS....spinach + kale + broccoli
fennel + lettuce + cabbage + sprouts
coconut water + herbals teas
hibiscus + camomile + aloe vera water
basil & other fresh herbs & roots etc
increasing hydration increases the
flow, so cleanses the cells

SMOOTHIES
heavy metal detox smoothies
frozen red berries
gluten free oats + chia seeds
pumpkin seeds + flax seeds
soaked almonds + other nuts
spices + roots + ashwagandha
goji berries + coconut water
avocado + coconut + fruits
coconut milk + spinach
black strap molasses
kale + spices + roots
leafy greens
sea weeds + dulce etc

PATHOGENS + TOXICITIES
viruses + bacteria + fungi
yeasts + candida + Mold
parasites + heavy metals
chemicals + farming + foods
water + air + personal products
furniture + clothes + perfume
candles + pharmaceuticals
avoid as much as you can
house hold sprays + cleaners
cooking in tin foil + non-stick pans
lead in paint + petrol + pipes etc
mercury in fish etc
chemicals in caffeine-free coffee

WEAN OFF
eggs + dairy + sugar
sweeteners + grains
alcohol + coffee
black tea + fizzy drinks
pork + soy + vinegar
fermented foods
milk chocolate
pastry + bread
rice + pasta
man-made foods
squash
muesli + granola
food in tins + jars

HEALING + SUPPLEMENTS
Holistic Healing for Mind, Body, and Spirit:
Achieving optimal health requires a multi-faceted approach that nurtures all aspects of our well-being. Incorporating a variety of methods can enhance healing, support recovery, and create lasting vitality. Some of the powerful practices and elements to integrate into your wellness routine include:
Mind-Body Practices:
Yoga and Breathwork to promote relaxation, flexibility, and balance.
Sound Healing (528Hz frequency) to support emotional and physical healing.
Poetry, Painting, and Journaling for emotional expression and stress release.
Counselling and Meditation for mental clarity and emotional processing.
Physical Detox and Restoration:
Massage, Sauna, Steam, and Swimming to detoxify and promote circulation.
Walking and Exercise to improve cardiovascular health and energy.
Castor Oil Packs to support liver detoxification.
Hydration and Rest are essential for rejuvenating your body and mind.

Nutrition and Healing Foods:
Juicing, Smoothies, and Soups rich in fresh fruits, vegetables, and healing herbs.
Spices, Fresh Herbs, and Roots (e.g., turmeric, ginger, garlic) to promote digestive health and inflammation reduction.
Vitamin C, D, B12, and Zinc to support immune function and overall health.
Nutrient-rich foods like Spirulina, Barley Grass Juice Powder, Atlantic Dulse, and Chaga Mushrooms to boost energy and detoxify.
Omega-3 Oils, Black Seed Oil, Milk Thistle, and Glutathione to promote liver health and fight oxidative stress.
Herbal Supplements for Wellness:
Lemon Balm, Echinacea, Cats' Claw, Elderberry, and Goldenseal for immunity and relaxation.
Ashwagandha, Ginseng, and Liquorice for stress relief and adrenal support.
NAC (N-Acetyl Cysteine) and CBD Oil for detoxification and mental clarity.
Probiotics and Digestive Enzymes to support gut health and digestion.
Natural Sweeteners & Nutritional Support:
Real Honey and Real Maple Syrup for a healthy energy boost.
Q10, L-Lysine, Turmeric, and GABA for cellular health and brain function.
Hibiscus, Camomile, Rose Hip, and Astaxanthin in herbal teas to support inflammation and relaxation.
By embracing this comprehensive, holistic approach, you can rejuvenate your mind and body, detoxify, nourish, and restore balance. Whether you're addressing specific health concerns or simply striving for improved overall wellness, consistency is key. Small, daily choices create lasting results, helping you thrive in a modern world full of challenges.

The Daily Cleansing choices + Healing Protocol
Healing Recipes and Daily Nourishment for Wellness:
1. **Hydration and Warm Beverages**:
    - **Lemon Water** or **Ginger Water** to kick-start digestion and boost energy.
    - **Thyme Tea** or your choice of real herbal tea (e.g., chamomile, peppermint), with **real honey** or **real maple syrup** for sweetness.
    - **Celery Juice**: Start with ½ cup and gradually increase to a pint per day over two weeks for detoxification and digestive support.
2. **Homemade Fruit Sauces and Smoothies**:
    - **Homemade Apple and Pear Sauce** with warming spices like **cinnamon, cloves, nutmeg**, or fresh **ginger** for a natural, comforting treat.
    - **Heavy Metal Detox Smoothie**:
        - 1 cup **blueberries**
        - 1 or 2 **bananas**
        - Juice of 1 or 2 **oranges**
        - ½ cup **coriander**
        - 1 tsp **spirulina**
        - 1 tsp **Atlantic Dulse**
        - 1 tsp **barley grass juice powder**

3. **Nourishing Meals and Soups:**
   - **Salad** with **avocado, leafy greens, asparagus, garlic,** and your choice of additional veggies, topped with a **homemade dressing**.
   - **Roasted Vegetable Soup**: A warming, nutrient-packed soup made with **butternut squash, sweet potatoes,** and spiced with **medjool dates** and **coconut water**.
   - **Hot Pots, Tray Bakes, and Soups** for comforting meals that provide deep nourishment.
   - **Lynn's Homemade Fruit Crumble**: A delicious, warming dessert with **GF oats, maple syrup or honey, medjool dates,** and a bit of **dark chocolate**.
4. **Sweet Treats and Snacks:**
   - **Lynn's Homemade Hot Chocolate:**
     - 1 **medjool date**
     - 1 tsp **GF oats**
     - 1 square of **85% dark chocolate**
     - **Water**
     - A pinch of **cinnamon**
     - **Real maple syrup** or **real honey** for sweetness.
   - **Lynn's Homemade Flapjacks**: Made with **GF oats, maple syrup or honey, medjool dates,** and a bit of **dark chocolate** for a wholesome snack.
5. **Everyday Healing Ingredients:**
   - **Fresh Herbs and Spices**: Include **ginger, garlic, turmeric,** and **fresh herbs** (e.g., basil, parsley) in your meals for natural anti-inflammatory and immune-boosting properties.
   - Healthy fats from **coconut oil** and **olive oil** for cooking and dressings.
   - **Juicing and Smoothies**: Enjoy nutrient-dense juices and smoothies, including **carrots, oranges, turmeric,** and **ginger** for detoxification and vitality.

Our lymphatic system acts as the body's waste disposal system, but it can become stagnant, toxic, pathogen-filled, and congested if not properly maintained. To support its function and detoxification, incorporating juicing with fresh herbs, green detox smoothies, and alkaline foods and drinks can help cleanse and flush out the lymphatic system and improve digestion.

The gut microbiome, which makes up 80% of our immune system, plays a crucial role in our overall health. By restoring and cleansing the gut, we can also support the liver, lymphatic system, and help to calm the adrenals and kidneys. Fresh herbs, spices, and roots possess powerful antimicrobial, antiviral, and antibacterial properties that help combat pathogens in the body. Over time, juicing and smoothies, enriched with green detox powders, can support the body in chelating toxins and promoting overall health.

Inflammation is often the result of an overload of pathogens and toxins, leading to a compromised body. REDOX imbalance occurs when there are too many free radicals and not enough antioxidants, causing oxidative stress at the cellular level. Combat this imbalance by focusing on a diet rich in raw, alkaline foods that nourish and restore the body.

All about Crohn's and colitis and IBD and celiac [there are 73,252 papers on Crohn's + 104,705 on colitis + 41,876 on celiac on pubmed.com]

IBS (Irritable Bowel Syndrome) is often linked to gut dysbiosis, bacterial biofilms, pathogens, inflammation, and stress.

Crohn's Disease is associated with pathogens, viruses, and inflammation.

Colitis typically involves pathogens, bacteria, viruses, gut dysbiosis, inflammation, and redox imbalance/oxidative stress.

Celiac Disease is linked to SIBO (Small Intestinal Bacterial Overgrowth), translocation of bacteria, pathogens, toxicities, and gut dysbiosis.

IBD (Inflammatory Bowel Disease) is primarily caused by gut dysbiosis, pathogens, oxidative stress, and inflammation.

Biofilms, which are colonies of bacteria and viruses, can thrive when the gut microbiome is disrupted. This disruption may occur due to factors like antibiotic use, an unhealthy diet, exposure to pathogens, or chemical toxicities in our environment or homes. Once these biofilms take hold, they can trick the immune system, causing it to go into overdrive in an attempt to eliminate them. To address this, fresh herbs can help eliminate the infection and break down the bacterial biofilms housed within the small intestine and bowel walls.

Juicing is an effective way to target and eliminate these invaders. Smoothies, too, are a better option, as they provide nourishment while aiding in healing. On the flip side, foods that feed pathogens, such as eggs, dairy, grains, sugar, pork, high-fat meals, and drinks like coffee, soda, and alcohol, must be addressed for healing to occur.

Healing the gut lining and cleansing the body of invaders is a gradual process that requires dedication. Diet alone doesn't cause these conditions, but it plays a crucial role in the healing journey. Weaning off harmful foods and incorporating healing meals and drinks takes time, practice, and a mindful approach to shopping and social situations. Patience and consistency are key.

Detox + Cleanse
1 Lemon water or ginger water
2 Celery juice or cucumber + apple
3 Heavy metal detox smoothie
1 banana + juice 1 orange +
Detox powder = Atlantic dulce +
Spirulina + barley grass juice powder
½ cup of coriander + cup of blueberries
4 avocado + asparagus salad etc
5 fresh herbs + spices + roots
6 ginger + turmeric + garlic
7 real honey + real maple syrup
8 veg tray bakes + hot pots
9 olive oil + coconut oil sparingly
10 dark chocolate 85% + medjool dates
11 home-made apple + pear sauce
12 soups + salads + smoothies + juicing

JUICING
celery [build slowly up to a pint a day]
1 cucumber + 2 apples or 2 pears + mint
2 oranges + 7 carrots + ginger + turmeric
1 cucumber + 1 head celery + 1 lemon
4 apples + [parsley or coriander]
1 courgette + 2 apples + cucumber
EXTRAS....spinach + kale + broccoli
fennel + lettuce + cabbage + sprouts
coconut water + herbals teas
hibiscus + camomile + aloe vera water
basil & other fresh herbs & roots etc
increasing hydration increases the
flow, so cleanses the cells

SMOOTHIES	**PATHOGENS + TOXICITIES**	**WEAN OFF**
heavy metal detox smoothies	viruses + bacteria + fungi	eggs + dairy + sugar
frozen red berries	yeasts + candida + Mold	sweeteners + grains
gluten free oats + chia seeds	parasites + heavy metals	alcohol + coffee
pumpkin seeds + flax seeds	chemicals + farming + foods	black tea + fizzy drinks
soaked almonds + other nuts	water + air + personal products	pork + soy + vinegar
spices + roots + ashwagandha	furniture + clothes + perfume	fermented foods
goji berries + coconut water	candles + pharmaceuticals	milk chocolate
avocado + coconut + fruits	avoid as much as you can	pastry + bread
coconut milk + spinach	house hold sprays + cleaners	rice + pasta
black strap molasses	cooking in tin foil + non-stick pans	man-made foods
kale + spices + roots	lead in paint + petrol + pipes etc	squash
leafy greens	mercury in fish etc	muesli + granola
sea weeds + dulce etc	chemicals in caffeine-free coffee	food in tins + jars

HEALING + SUPPLEMENTS

Holistic Healing Approach:
Nutrition & Detoxification:
Eating and drinking little and often
Juicing, smoothies, salads, soups, and vegetables
Nutrients: Vitamin C, D, B12, Zinc, Spirulina, Barley Grass Juice Powder, Atlantic Dulce, Chaga Mushrooms, Turmeric, Ginger, Garlic, Cat's Claw, Echinacea, Elderberry, Blackstrap Molasses, Omega-3 Oils, Ginseng, Kelp, Black Seed Oil, Liquorice, L-Lysine, GABA, Coenzyme Q10 (Q10), Glutathione, Milk Thistle
Fresh herbs, spices, and roots (e.g., turmeric, ginger, garlic, cinnamon)
Herbal teas: Hibiscus, Chamomile, Rose Hip, Oregano Oil, Black Walnut Hulls
Mind-Body Practices:
Yoga, including handstand stool practice
Breathwork
Sound healing at 528Hz
Rebounding (mini-trampoline exercises)
Walking and Swimming
Restorative Therapies:
Essential oils (via diffuser)
Baths (detoxifying with Epsom salts, herbs, etc.)
Massage, Sauna, Steam
Castor oil packs
Emotional and Psychological Support:
Journaling
Poetry and Painting for self-expression
Counselling and Therapy
Change of environment: Job, home, relationships
Other Supporting Practices:
Hydration (drink plenty of water)
Rest, Relaxation, and Sleep
Prebiotics, Probiotics, and Digestive Enzymes

Adaptogens like Ashwagandha and CBD oil
NAC (N-acetyl cysteine)
Superfoods & Supplements:
Spirulina, Barley Grass Juice Powder
Omega-3 oils, Turmeric, Ginger, and Garlic
Zinc, Vitamin C, D, and B12
Probiotic-rich foods and supplements

The Daily Cleansing choices + Healing Protocol

Hydrating & Detoxifying Drinks:
Lemon or Ginger Water: Add fresh lemon or ginger slices to warm water for a soothing, detoxifying drink. You can also sweeten with real honey or maple syrup.
Herbal Tea: Choose your preferred herbal tea, and sweeten naturally with honey or maple syrup.
Celery Juice: Start with ½ cup and gradually build up to 1 pint per day over two weeks to support digestion and detox.
Ginger and Thyme Water: Combine fresh ginger and thyme in warm water, adding honey or maple syrup for sweetness.

Healthy, Nourishing Recipes:
Homemade Apple & Pear Sauce: A simple, spiced treat with cinnamon, cloves, nutmeg, or real ginger for flavour.

Juicing Recipe:
5 carrots
2 oranges
1 tsp real turmeric
1-inch piece of fresh ginger
This combination provides a nutrient-packed, anti-inflammatory juice.

Heavy Metal Detox Smoothie:
1 cup of blueberries
1 or 2 bananas
Juice of 1 or 2 oranges
½ cup coriander
1 tsp spirulina
1 tsp Atlantic Dulce
1 tsp barley grass juice powder
This smoothie helps detoxify heavy metals and nourish the body.

Salads:
A vibrant salad made with avocado, leafy greens, asparagus, garlic, and any other fresh veggies you love. Top with a homemade dressing of your choice.
Roasted Vegetable Soup:
Use root vegetables like butternut squash and sweet potatoes for a hearty, flavourful soup. Add Medjool dates for natural sweetness and coconut water for a smooth texture.

Sweets & Comfort Foods:
Lynn's Homemade Hot Chocolate:
1 Medjool date
1 tsp gluten-free oats
1 square of 85% dark chocolate
Water
A sprinkle of cinnamon
Sweeten with real maple syrup or honey

This warming, nourishing drink is a perfect cozy treat.
Lynn's Homemade Flapjacks:
GF oats
Maple syrup or honey
Medjool dates
Dark chocolate
A wholesome, sweet snack with natural ingredients.
Lynn's Fruit Crumble:
A simple and delicious dessert made from fresh fruits, topped with a crispy, healthy crumble.

Meals to Nourish & Heal:
Hot Pots and Tray Bakes: Easy one-pot meals filled with vegetables and protein, baked together for comfort and nutrition.
Soups and Stews: Fill your soups with a variety of vegetables, roots, and spices for rich, healing Flavors.
Salads: Refreshing, nutrient-dense meals that can include a variety of vegetables, fruits, and healthy fats.
Smoothies & Juices: Perfect for quick, nutrient-dense meals or snacks, packed with fruits, vegetables, and detoxifying herbs and powders.

Healthy Ingredients:
Fruits & Vegetables: Fresh, seasonal produce, packed with vitamins and antioxidants.
Fresh Herbs & Spices: Ginger, garlic, turmeric, cinnamon, cloves, and other healing roots and spices.
Healthy Fats: Coconut oil and olive oil and avocado oil for cooking and dressings.

All about asthma and eczema and allergies [there are 229,266 papers on asthma + 27,096 on eczema + 608,673 on allergies on pubmed.com]
Asthma: Asthma is primarily driven by **inflammation** and **congestion**, with key contributing factors being:
Oxidative stress: This occurs when there are not enough antioxidants to counteract free radicals in the body. To address this, focus on a nutrient-rich diet and consider adding **buffered vitamin C powder** for its antioxidant properties.
Pathogens and toxicities: Yeast, bacteria, viruses, fungi, and parasites can all play a role in exacerbating asthma symptoms.
Chemical toxicities and heavy metals: These can act as triggers or root causes for asthma, so it's essential to minimize exposure to environmental toxins.
Eczema:
Eczema often reflects an imbalance in the body's detox processes:
Gut microbiome: Poor skin health is commonly linked to an unhealthy gut, often stemming from an imbalance in gut bacteria.
Sluggish liver: A congested or overloaded liver can affect skin health.
Pathogens and toxicities: Chemical exposure, dehydration, and infections can contribute to eczema flare-ups.

Allergies: Allergies are typically the result of high histamine levels, which are linked to gut microbiome imbalances, often caused by:

Pathogen infections: Bacteria, yeast, and other pathogens can trigger allergic reactions.

Dietary factors: A diet high in dairy, fats, sugar, and congesting grains can also worsen allergies.

Root Causes of These Conditions:

These three conditions—**asthma**, **eczema**, and **allergies**—are becoming more common due to increased **toxic exposures** from household chemicals, processed foods, and overuse of pharmaceuticals (such as antibiotics), which disrupt the microbiome and immune system.

Children are especially vulnerable to these threats and need more antioxidants, herbs, roots, and spices to support their health.

Dietary and Lifestyle Changes to Support Healing:

Juicing & Smoothies:

Fresh juices and smoothies are excellent for breakfast, providing essential nutrients to support the immune system and gut health. A great option is a **homemade apple and pear sauce** to reset the gut.

Dietary Modifications:

Focus on eliminating foods that exacerbate these conditions:

Dairy, **refined sugars**, **sweeteners** (watch for hidden sugars in packaged foods)

Gluten, wheat, eggs, pork, and **processed foods**

Avoid **fizzy drinks, pizza,** and **factory-made meals**.

Ancient Diets:

Diets like **paleo** (pre-farming, ancestral diets) tend to be the best option as they focus on whole, unprocessed foods that nourish the body without causing inflammation.

Smoothie and Juicing Tips for Kids:

Transitioning kids to a healthier diet can be difficult, so focus on simple swaps:

Start with **juicing apples, oranges, ginger, and turmeric**—children love fresh juices.

Gradually replace store-bought juices with fresh ones, as store-bought juices often lack enzymes and contain added sugars.

Avoid **nut milks** and **oat milks** (as they can be congesting for kids with constipation) and opt for **fresh, homemade options**.

Skin Care:

Use **aloe vera** on the skin to soothe eczema or irritation.

Avocados are rich in **vitamin E** and can be added to smoothies or eaten on their own to help support healthy skin.

Toxins and Household Changes:

Avoid chemical sprays, cleaners, and perfumes in the home.

Keep pets off furniture and beds to reduce allergens.

Use essential oils sparingly and try **steam inhalations** for respiratory support.

Little Changes Over Time:

It's important to make gradual, sustainable changes rather than trying to overhaul a child's diet all at once. Focus on easy-to-implement changes like **juicing** and swapping store-bought snacks with healthier homemade options (e.g., **flapjacks** made with Medjool dates, real honey, and maple syrup).

Conclusion:
Improving your child's diet and lifestyle requires **patience** and **consistency**. Start with small, manageable changes and gradually increase the number of healthy foods and practices. Over time, these adjustments will help address the root causes of asthma, eczema, and allergies, allowing the body to heal naturally.

Detox + Cleanse
1 Lemon water or ginger water
2 Celery juice or cucumber + apple
3 Heavy metal detox smoothie
1 banana + juice 1 orange +
Detox powder = Atlantic dulce +
Spirulina + barley grass juice powder
½ cup of coriander + cup of blueberries
4 avocado + asparagus salad etc
5 fresh herbs + spices + roots
6 ginger + turmeric + garlic
7 real honey + real maple syrup
8 veg tray bakes + hot pots
9 olive oil + coconut oil sparingly
10 dark chocolate 85% + medjool dates
11 home-made apple + pear sauce
12 soups + salads + smoothies + juicing

JUICING
celery [build slowly up to a pint a day]
1 cucumber + 2 apples or 2 pears + mint
2 oranges + 7 carrots + ginger + turmeric
1 cucumber + 1 head celery + 1 lemon
4 apples + [parsley or coriander]
1 courgette + 2 apples + cucumber
EXTRAS....spinach + kale + broccoli
fennel + lettuce + cabbage + sprouts
coconut water + herbals teas
hibiscus + camomile + aloe vera water
basil & other fresh herbs & roots etc
increasing hydration increases the
flow, so cleanses the cells

SMOOTHIES
heavy metal detox smoothies
frozen red berries
gluten free oats + chia seeds
pumpkin seeds + flax seeds
soaked almonds + other nuts
spices + roots + ashwagandha
goji berries + coconut water
avocado + coconut + fruits
coconut milk + spinach
black strap molasses
kale + spices + roots
leafy greens
sea weeds + dulce etc

PATHOGENS + TOXICITIES
viruses + bacteria + fungi
yeasts + candida + Mold
parasites + heavy metals
chemicals + farming + foods
water + air + personal products
furniture + clothes + perfume
candles + pharmaceuticals
avoid as much as you can
house hold sprays + cleaners
cooking in tin foil + non-stick pans
lead in paint + petrol + pipes etc
mercury in fish etc
chemicals in caffeine-free coffee

WEAN OFF
eggs + dairy + sugar
sweeteners + grains
alcohol + coffee
black tea + fizzy drinks
pork + soy + vinegar
fermented foods
milk chocolate
pastry + bread
rice + pasta
man-made foods
squash
muesli + granola
food in tins + jars

HEALING + SUPPLEMENTS: Holistic Health Practices:
- **Nutrition & Detoxification:**
  A balanced diet rich in **whole foods**, fresh herbs, **roots**, and **spices** is essential for healing. Focus on nutrient-dense options like **juicing, smoothies, salads, soups,** and plenty of **vegetables**. Consider adding:
    - **Vitamin C, Vitamin D, B12, Zinc, Spirulina, Barley grass juice powder, Atlantic dulce,** and **Turmeric** for their anti-inflammatory properties.
    - **Fresh herbs** like **lemon balm, ginger, garlic, echinacea, elderberry,** and **cats' claw** help boost immunity and support overall health.

- - **Omega-3 oils, Black seed oil, Kelp, Ginseng,** and **Ashwagandha** provide anti-inflammatory, mood-boosting, and adaptogenic benefits.
- **Supplementation & Herbal Support:**
  Adding **chaga mushrooms, goldenseal, blackstrap molasses, liquorice, L-lysine, GABA, CoQ10, Glutathione, Milk thistle,** and **NAC (N-acetyl cysteine)** can support detoxification, liver health, and overall healing.
  Drink **herbal teas** like **hibiscus, chamomile, oregano oil,** and **rose hip** for soothing effects and immune support.
- **Lifestyle & Movement:** Incorporate **exercise** like **yoga, walking,** and **swimming** to keep the body active and release stress. Activities like **breathwork, rebounding, massage, sauna,** and **steam baths** support circulation, detoxification, and overall relaxation. Consider using a **handstand yoga stool** for additional stretching and strength.
- **Mental & Emotional Well-being:** Practices like **counselling, journaling,** and engaging in creative outlets such as **poetry** and **painting** can improve mental clarity and emotional balance.
  Use **sound healing** with frequencies like **528 Hz** to promote healing, and **essential oils** in a **diffuser** for calming, therapeutic effects.
- **Rest & Relaxation:**
  Prioritize **rest, relaxation,** and **sleep** for healing. Aim for **hydration** and eating smaller, more frequent meals throughout the day to maintain energy levels and avoid stress on your digestive system.
  Castor oil packs can support detoxification, while **baths** with Epsom salts or essential oils help soothe the body.
- **Natural Sweeteners:**
  Use **real honey** and **real maple syrup** as natural, unrefined sweeteners in your diet for their nutritional benefits.

By combining these practices, you can address multiple areas of health—nutrition, physical movement, emotional well-being, and detoxification—in a holistic way. This balanced approach supports long-term wellness and healing.

The Daily Cleansing choices + Healing Protocol
Morning Boosters:
Lemon Water or Ginger Water:
Start your day with a glass of warm lemon water or ginger water to hydrate and kickstart your digestion. Add thyme or a herbal tea of your choice for extra health benefits. Sweeten naturally with real honey or real maple syrup.
Homemade Apple & Pear Sauce:
A great gut-friendly meal! Add warming spices like cinnamon, cloves, nutmeg, or fresh ginger for an extra boost of flavour and health benefits.
Celery Juice:
Start with ½ cup of celery juice and gradually increase to 1 pint a day over 2 weeks. This helps cleanse the system and improve gut health.

Juicing & Smoothies:
- **Carrot & Orange Juice:**
Juice **5 carrots, 2 oranges**, and add **1 tsp of real turmeric** and a **1-inch piece of fresh ginger**. This antioxidant-packed juice supports your immune system and reduces inflammation.
- **Heavy Metal Detox Smoothie:**
    - 1 cup **blueberries**
    - 1-2 **bananas**
    - Juice of **1 or 2 oranges**
    - ½ cup **coriander**
    - 1 tsp **spirulina**
    - 1 tsp **Atlantic dulce**
    - 1 tsp **barley grass juice powder**

This nutrient-rich smoothie helps cleanse the body of toxins and supports liver health.

Meals & Soups:
- **Salads:**
A refreshing and nourishing salad with **avocado, leafy greens, asparagus, garlic,** and your choice of veggies. Top it with a **homemade dressing** for extra flavour.
- **Roasted Vegetable Soup:**
A hearty, warming soup made with **butternut squash, sweet potatoes, medjool dates,** and **coconut water** for a creamy texture.

Snack Ideas & Treats:
- **Lynn's Homemade Hot Chocolate:**
A cozy drink made with:
    - 1 **medjool date**
    - 1 tsp **gluten-free oats**
    - 1 square **85% dark chocolate**
    - Water
    - **Cinnamon**
    - **Real maple syrup** or **real honey**
- **Lynn's Homemade Flapjacks:**
Made with **gluten-free oats, maple syrup** or **honey, medjool dates,** and **dark chocolate**. These make a great, healthier alternative to store-bought sweet treats.
- **Fruit Crumble:**
A homemade **fruit crumble** using seasonal fruits, and a topping made with **gluten-free oats** and a touch of **maple syrup** or **honey**.

Meals for Healing:
- **Hot Pots & Tray Bakes:**
Nourishing one-pot meals and tray bakes that combine root vegetables like **sweet potatoes, carrots,** and **onions**, along with lean proteins if desired, all baked together for an easy, comforting meal.
- **Soups:**
Always a good option for comfort and nourishment. opt for a variety of vegetable-based soups that include fresh herbs, **roots** (like **ginger, garlic,** and **turmeric**), and anti-inflammatory ingredients.

Healthy Fats & Cooking Oils:
- Use **coconut oil** or **olive oil** in cooking for their anti-inflammatory and heart-healthy properties.

By focusing on these nutrient-dense meals and drinks, you can easily support your body's healing process with wholesome, detoxifying foods. Each component is designed to boost immunity, reduce inflammation, and support gut health.

Medicinal Herbs + Spices + Roots + health benefits [pubmed.com]

All fresh herbs + spices + roots have potent medical properties, anti-pathogen, anti-inflammatory and anti-parasitic. Try to use some every day, either in cooking, a salad or A herbal broth when ill or just A herbal tea first thing in the morning.

Fresh herbs are best, fresh roots are best, but we can have powdered or oils or dried or capsules in place of fresh. Always take as a course and not all the time, always check for any interactions with your health care provider.

Garlic is anti-viral, anti-fungal, anti-bacterial, anti-parasitic, anti-cancer, boosts the immune system, anti-inflammatory, antioxidant, helps rid heavy metals, good for all chronic health conditions and colds and flu in broths cooked, or raw,

Ginger is a pain killer for joints and stomach and women's menstrual cramps, anti-inflammatory, anti-cancer, anti-pathogen, make into a tea, or blend with water and strain or use in a juicer, good for sore throats + headaches, the fresh root is best, fights viruses, cleans arteries, aids weight loss, anti-viral,

Turmeric is anti-inflammatory, fights pathogens, anti-cancer, pain killer for joints, lowers cholesterol, helps rid heavy metals, use in cooking or in a juicer, the fresh root is best,

Parsley is a great body alkaliser, anti-pathogen, freshens breath, supports the bladder, improves kidneys, blood cleanser, improves lymphatic drainage,

Coriander pulls out heavy metals, detoxes the liver, fights viruses, supports the adrenals, anti-parasitic, use in soups and fresh juicers, anti-pathogen,

Mustard seed anti-pathogen, antioxidant, anti-inflammatory,

Rosemary, sage, thyme, the aromatic herbs, easy to grow and great for all cooking, can be juiced in small quantities, thyme tea is a great cold and flu remedy, rosemary aids oestrogen balance, great for dementia, Alzheimer's, sage is an anti-septic,

Cinnamon is anti-pathogen, anti-tumour, antioxidant, cholesterol lowering, helps with blood sugar control, heart health + arteries,

Cloves are a painkiller, antibacterial, antibacterial activities, antifungal, anticancer, antioxidant, cleans arteries

Herbal teas, Chamomile, Hibiscus, Peppermint, Thyme, Lemon, Ginger etc [can add real honey or real maples syrup]

Astaxanthin is powerful antioxidant, the highest one,

Oregano oil a potent anti-bacterial killer, anti-biotic, anti-parasite, etc, only takes as a course and never all the time

Barley grass juice powder, spirulina, Atlantic dulce, all round health aids, are all-round health supporters, high in nutrition and have abilities to cleanse organs and support healing,

Cardamon potent anti-inflammatory, anti-pathogen, antioxidant,

Ginseng all round health supporter, immune supporter,

Lemon balm calms nerves so great for depression, anxiety, bipolar, sleep issues, a relaxant

Nutmeg use sparingly, not a tsp every day, aids appetite, cholesterol lowering, digestive aid, sleep aid,

Cayenne pepper improves blood flow, great for heart health + angina, reduces plague in arteries, aids digestion, helps with weight loss,

Ashwagandha calms the adrenals down, stress buster, great for mental health, anxiety, depression, bipolar, sleep aid, thyroid aid, immune booster,

Paprika improves circulation, blood pressure, anti-pathogen,

Star anise immune booster, heart health, blood + cholesterol, anti-pathogen, kills bacteria,

Basil cardio-protection, antioxidant and antimicrobial effects, and anti-inflammatory, antiulcer, anticoagulant, and anti-depressant properties,

Peppermint great for cognitive brain health, dental health, urinary retention, skin and wound healing, anti-depressant, anti-anxiety effects, calms stomach nerves, stomach gas, pain killer,

Black Cumin seed oil, protects the heart + brain, cancer, reproductive aid, cancer aid, fights oxidative stress, respiratory aid, kidney aid,

Mushrooms, shitake, chaga, lions mane, cordyceps, reishi, anti-diabetic, antioxidant, antimicrobial, anticancer, prebiotic, immunomodulating, anti-inflammatory and cardiovascular benefits,

Ginkgo biloba has been shown in trials to help with Alzheimer's + dementia, it improves blood flow, anti-inflammatory, thins sticky thick blood, an antioxidant.

All about long covid and chronic fatigue syndrome and fibromyalgia [there are 37,058 papers on long covid + 11,335 on CFS + 15,284 on fibromyalgia on pubmed.com]

ME + CFS (Myalgic Encephalomyelitis / Chronic Fatigue Syndrome):

chronic fatigue syndrome (CFS) often stems from post-viral illness, where the body's immune system becomes overwhelmed due to pathogens that trigger ongoing immune activation, much like in autoimmune conditions. This persistent immune response leads to cellular damage, particularly to the mitochondria, the energy powerhouses of our cells. The oxidative stress from this continuous activation disrupts normal redox processes, resulting in fatigue, malaise, and an inability to generate sufficient energy.

This condition also significantly affects gut mobility and digestion, making it difficult for the body to absorb nutrients properly. As a result, people with CFS may struggle with poor digestion and nutrition, which further compounds the cycle of fatigue.

The Progression of CFS

Like most chronic diseases, CFS tends to progress in stages. The goal in healing is to address the underlying causes, restore mitochondrial function, and break the cycle of immune overactivation. Healing from CFS requires a comprehensive approach, and while the exact protocol may vary depending on the stage of the illness, there are common strategies that can support recovery:

Key Healing Protocols for CFS:

1. **Antiviral Protocols:**
   Given that viral pathogens often play a central role in CFS, following a targeted antiviral protocol is essential to reduce viral load, eliminate infections, and support immune function. This protocol should focus on eradicating pathogens while simultaneously supporting the body's healing processes.

2. **Gut Health:**
   As CFS affects digestion, it's crucial to focus on gut healing. Juicing and smoothies, which are easier to digest and absorb, are a great way to provide nourishment while reducing the digestive load. Fresh, homemade juices can be packed with vitamins and antioxidants that support mitochondrial function and overall immune health. Aim to build up to 1 litre or more of fresh juice daily to super hydrate and provide liquid nutrition that accelerates healing.

3. **Nutrient-Rich Foods:**
   Soft fruits, particularly when warmed and made into a sauce, are an excellent option for CFS sufferers. These can be enhanced with healing spices (such as ginger, turmeric, and garlic) and roots that help combat pathogens and support detoxification. Regular intake of these foods will not only support digestion but also promote the elimination of viruses and toxins from the body.

The Role of Diet in Healing:

- Transitioning to a healing dietary protocol is essential to give the body the nutrients it needs to recover. The shift requires time, patience, and a careful approach, especially when the patient may be bedridden. In these cases, it's often the responsibility of the caregiver to support the healing process through diet and lifestyle changes.

- **Avoiding Harmful Foods:**
  Reducing or eliminating foods that aggravate inflammation, such as processed sugars, gluten, dairy, and refined grains, is crucial in easing digestive strain and reducing immune activation. The goal is to replace these with nutrient-dense, anti-inflammatory foods that support healing.
- **The Dangers of Pathogen Resistance:**
  Pathogens can develop resistance to antibiotics over time, which can make treatment more challenging and lead to further digestive complications. A carefully designed protocol that includes not just antiviral treatments, but also nutritional support can help break this cycle.

Understanding the Modern World of Superbugs:
In today's world, the presence of super bacteria and super viruses is a growing concern. These pathogens can evade the body's defences, overwhelming the immune system and triggering chronic conditions like CFS. The immune system, already under strain, becomes less capable of combating infections, which makes comprehensive healing protocols essential for recovery.

An "Everything in Moderation" Approach Isn't Enough:
Given the complexities of CFS and its connection to chronic immune activation, a traditional "everything in moderation" approach will not be sufficient for tackling the underlying issues. To recover from CFS, a well-rounded, specialized healing protocol is necessary—one that addresses viral load, mitochondrial health, gut function, and immune support.
This protocol requires a focused approach, consistent effort, and a mindset dedicated to long-term recovery. With the right support, diet, and healing strategies, progress is possible.

Detox + Cleanse
1 Lemon water or ginger water
2 Celery juice or cucumber + apple
3 Heavy metal detox smoothie
1 banana + juice 1 orange +
Detox powder = Atlantic dulce +
Spirulina + barley grass juice powder
½ cup of coriander + cup of blueberries
4 avocado + asparagus salad etc
5 fresh herbs + spices + roots
6 ginger + turmeric + garlic
7 real honey + real maple syrup
8 veg tray bakes + hot pots
9 olive oil + coconut oil sparingly
10 dark chocolate 85% + medjool dates
11 home-made apple + pear sauce
12 soups + salads + smoothies + juicing

JUICING
celery [build slowly up to a pint a day]
1 cucumber + 2 apples or 2 pears + mint
2 oranges + 7 carrots + ginger + turmeric
1 cucumber + 1 head celery + 1 lemon
4 apples + [parsley or coriander]
1 courgette + 2 apples + cucumber
EXTRAS....spinach + kale + broccoli
fennel + lettuce + cabbage + sprouts
coconut water + herbals teas
hibiscus + camomile + aloe vera water
basil & other fresh herbs & roots etc
increasing hydration increases the
flow, so cleanses the cells

SMOOTHIES	PATHOGENS + TOXICITIES	WEAN OFF
heavy metal detox smoothies	viruses + bacteria + fungi	eggs + dairy + sugar
frozen red berries	yeasts + candida + Mold	sweeteners + grains
gluten free oats + chia seeds	parasites + heavy metals	alcohol + coffee
pumpkin seeds + flax seeds	chemicals + farming + foods	black tea + fizzy drinks
soaked almonds + other nuts	water + air + personal products	pork + soy + vinegar
spices + roots + ashwagandha	furniture + clothes + perfume	fermented foods
goji berries + coconut water	candles + pharmaceuticals	milk chocolate
avocado + coconut + fruits	avoid as much as you can	pastry + bread
coconut milk + spinach	house hold sprays + cleaners	rice + pasta
black strap molasses	cooking in tin foil + non-stick pans	man-made foods
kale + spices + roots	lead in paint + petrol + pipes etc	squash
leafy greens	mercury in fish etc	muesli + granola
sea weeds + dulce etc	chemicals in caffeine-free coffee	food in tins + jars

HEALING + SUPPLEMENTS

Holistic Healing Approach for Mind, Body, and Spirit

To foster overall well-being and healing, a multifaceted approach combining nutrition, detoxification, and self-care practices is essential. This comprehensive plan addresses physical, emotional, and spiritual health. Here are the key components:

1. Nutrition & Detoxification

A healing diet is crucial for restoring balance. Prioritize the following:

Fruits & Vegetables: Fresh juices, smoothies, salads, soups, and vegetables are essential for nourishment.

Healing Herbs & Roots: Incorporate turmeric, ginger, garlic, cinnamon, cloves, and fresh herbs for their anti-inflammatory and detoxifying properties.

Spices: Include powerful spices like turmeric, ginger, and garlic to support digestion and immune health.

Superfoods & Supplements:

Vitamin C & D
B12
Zinc
Spirulina
Barley Grass Juice Powder
Atlantic Dulce
Chaga Mushrooms
Elderberry
Goldenseal
Ashwagandha
Ginseng
Omega-3 Oils
Probiotics & Prebiotics
Digestive Enzymes
Milk Thistle
Blackstrap Molasses
NAC (N-acetyl cysteine)
CBD Oil
L-Lysine

Glutathione
CoQ10
Liquorice
Black Seed Oil
Astaxanthin
Rose Hip
Lemon Balm
Oregano Oil
Hibiscus
Camomile
Black Walnut Hulls
Real Honey & Maple Syrup (for natural sweetness)

2. Movement & Exercise

Incorporating regular movement into your day is essential for both physical and mental well-being:

Yoga & Breathwork: Practices such as yoga and breathwork help relax the nervous system, reduce stress, and enhance circulation. Consider adding sound healing with 528 Hz frequency for deep cellular healing.

Walking & Swimming: Low-impact exercises that promote circulation and overall vitality.

Rebounding: A fun way to improve lymphatic drainage and support detoxification.

Handstand Yoga Stool: For those looking to deepen their practice and engage the upper body and core.

3. Stress Reduction & Self-Care

Managing stress is a critical aspect of healing, and these practices support relaxation and balance:

Massage: Regular massages to relax muscles, relieve tension, and improve circulation.

Sauna & Steam: Help detoxify the body, improve skin health, and relax muscles.

Essential Oils & Diffusers: Use oils such as lavender, eucalyptus, or frankincense to promote relaxation and alleviate stress.

Sound Healing: Listen to healing frequencies like 528 Hz to aid in emotional and physical healing.

Hot Baths: Soak in warm baths to reduce muscle tension and promote detoxification.

4. Emotional & Mental Well-being

Supporting mental and emotional health is essential for healing:

Poetry & Painting: Creative activities to express emotions and foster mindfulness.

Counselling: Professional therapy can help process emotions and release past trauma.

Journaling: A powerful tool for reflection, emotional release, and self-awareness.

5. Rest, Hydration & Sleep

Restful sleep, hydration, and relaxation are key to rejuvenating the body:

Rest & Relaxation: Ensure adequate rest to allow your body to heal and regenerate.

Hydration: Drink plenty of water, herbal teas, and fresh juices throughout the day.

Sleep: Prioritize good sleep hygiene to support the body's natural healing processes.

6. Lifestyle & Environment

Creating a supportive environment can amplify your healing journey:

Change in Environment: Consider adjusting your work, home, and relationships to reduce stress and create a healing space.

Castor Oil Packs: Excellent for detoxification and supporting organ health.

Natural Products: Use natural cleaning products, essential oils, and fabrics to minimize chemical exposure.

By integrating these practices, you create a nurturing, supportive foundation for healing and self-care. Combining these holistic approaches helps bring balance to the body, mind, and spirit, fostering optimal well-being and vitality.

The Daily Cleansing choices + Healing Protocol
Nutrient-Dense and Healing Recipes
Hydrating and Healing Beverages
- **Lemon Water / Ginger Water:** Start the day with a hydrating, detoxifying beverage.
- **Herbal Tea:** Choose from thyme, chamomile, peppermint, or any herbal tea of your choice. Add real honey or real maple syrup for natural sweetness.
- **Apple & Pear Sauce:** Homemade with a blend of cinnamon, cloves, nutmeg, or fresh ginger for extra flavour and warmth.
- **Celery Juice:** Start with ½ a cup and gradually increase to 1 pint daily over 2 weeks to support detoxification and digestion.

Fresh Juices & Smoothies
- **Carrot & Orange Juice:** Blend 5 carrots, 2 oranges, 1 tsp of real turmeric, and 1-inch of fresh ginger for a refreshing and anti-inflammatory drink.
- **Heavy Metal Detox Smoothie:**
    - 1 cup of blueberries
    - 1 or 2 bananas
    - Juice of 1 or 2 oranges
    - ½ cup fresh coriander
    - 1 tsp spirulina
    - 1 tsp Atlantic dulce
    - 1 tsp barley grass juice powder
    - Blend all ingredients for a nourishing, detoxifying boost.

Nourishing Meals
- **Avocado Salad:** Fresh leafy greens, avocado, asparagus, garlic, and your favorite salad ingredients topped with a homemade dressing.
- **Roasted Veg Soup:** A warming bowl of butternut squash and sweet potatoes, perfect for cold weather. Add a handful of medjool dates and coconut water for extra flavour and sweetness.

Comforting Treats
- **Lynn's Homemade Hot Chocolate:**
    - 1 medjool date
    - 1 tsp gluten-free oats
    - 1 square of 85% dark chocolate
    - Water, cinnamon, and either real maple syrup or honey for a sweet touch.
- **Lynn's Homemade Flapjacks:**
    - Gluten-free oats
    - Maple syrup or honey
    - Medjool dates
    - Dark chocolate chunks
    - A satisfying, wholesome snack.
- **Lynn's Fruit Crumble:** A comforting dessert with seasonal fruit, topped with a crumbly, gluten-free oat topping.

Hearty and Wholesome Meals
- **Hot Pots & Tray Bakes:** A comforting and filling meal, perfect for nourishing your body with vegetables and protein.
- **Soups & Stews:** Packed with vegetables like carrots, sweet potatoes, butternut squash, and garlic, along with herbs and spices for added flavour and healing properties.

Everyday Essentials
- **Salads:** Consistently incorporate salads into your meals for raw, fresh nutrients. Top with healthy fats like avocado or olive oil.
- **Juicing & Smoothies:** Keep up with daily juicing and smoothies to ensure you're getting enough vitamins and minerals from fresh produce. Add fresh herbs like ginger, garlic, and turmeric to enhance their healing properties.

Healthy Fats & Oils
- **Coconut Oil:** Great for cooking or adding to smoothies for a healthy fat boost.
- **Olive Oil:** Use for dressings or drizzling over salads to add healthy fats and antioxidants.
-

All about the KETO diet, the low carb diet and neurological inflammation

High Carbohydrate Diets and Neurological Health

High carbohydrate intake can fuel inflammation, which has significant impacts on brain health, potentially contributing to conditions like dementia, Alzheimer's, epilepsy, autism, ADHD, and other mental health issues. In these cases, a low-carb or even a ketogenic (keto) diet may be necessary. A keto diet, specifically, is a super low-carb approach that may help address these concerns.

Neurological inflammation is often linked to gut inflammation. When the gut microbiome becomes imbalanced—due to factors such as poor diet, pathogens, bacteria, parasites, stress, high cortisol levels, toxins, etc.—inflammatory cytokines can travel to the brain. If this happens for an extended period, it can lead to increased permeability of the blood-brain barrier, creating a chronic, harmful cycle that negatively affects both brain and overall health.

If this process is understood and addressed early, when a condition is first diagnosed, achieving remission or even reversal is possible. A low-carb or keto diet should be explored as part of the healing protocol. While transitioning to a keto diet can be effective, it's often preferable to make a gradual switch, rather than abruptly changing to a radically different diet.

This is a vast topic that warrants further study, and I encourage you to explore it in more depth to better understand how these dietary changes can impact neurological health.

Starting a Low-Carb/Keto Diet for Healing

To begin a low-carb or keto diet, it's essential to create a plan outlining all the foods and habits that need to be swapped. There are over 6,000 studies on keto available on PubMed.com, so if you're interested in diving deeper, that's a great place to start. However, there are only a few hundred studies focusing on keto for conditions like dementia, autism, and mental health, as this area remains under-researched. Unfortunately, pharmaceutical companies are more inclined to study medications because they are highly profitable, whereas natural healing pathways like keto are less lucrative.

Nonetheless, I have personally studied and used the keto diet to reclaim my health and address neurological issues. Chronic brain and mental health disorders are rising, but it's important to recognize that much of this is due to our toxic environments—chemicals in our homes, pesticides in food and water, and industrial food production. While these factors contribute, it's crucial not to dwell on them. Instead, we must focus our energy on healing.

The key is to gather what we need for healing, bring it into our homes, and commit to the practice of recovery every day. This means preparing nourishing meals, resting, and exercising when we feel strong enough. The keto diet can help calm our minds, reduce inflammation, eliminate toxins and pathogens, and ultimately improve our well-being.

By following this healing path, we can lift brain fog, restore our energy, and regain clarity of thought. This is the reclamation of our minds and our health.

Starting a Keto (Low-Carb) Diet

I've outlined a simple guide to help you transition to a keto diet. While there are many acceptable foods on a keto diet, it's important to focus on what works for you and take your time. There's no rush—gradually swapping out high-carb foods over a few days or weeks is the way to go.

The highest sources of carbohydrates are sugary puddings, cakes, and grains. The keto diet is similar to the Paleo diet, which focuses on foods from before the era of large-scale farming, specifically the cultivation of wheat. Many people find that gluten is an inflammatory agent, and grains in general can contribute to inflammation, particularly for those with chronic illnesses. Personally, I've chosen to live grain-free, even though it was challenging at first (giving up bread and rice). Now, I feel much better for it.

I rely on vegetables as my primary carbohydrate source, and as you can see from my recipes, I love sweet potatoes. While sweet potatoes are not strictly keto, they're still a good option when balanced with the rest of your plan. The key is finding what works for you—whether you choose to include some carbs or keep them limited.

As you make this transition, gradually reduce the problematic foods like dairy, eggs, and grains. Most of my recipes are low-carb, and the goal is to focus on the entire day's meals, not just individual ones. It takes time for your body to adjust to burning ketones instead of glucose, so be patient with the process. Remember, this isn't a quick fix, but a long-term lifestyle change for better health.

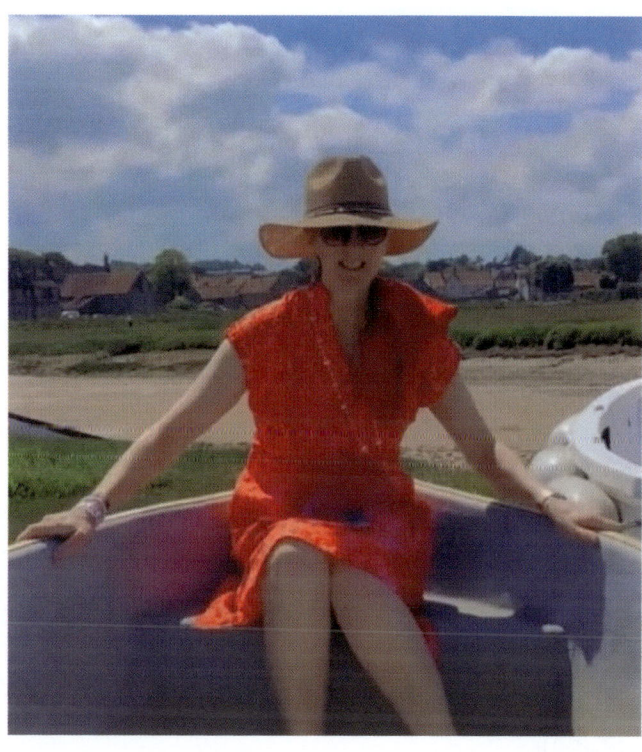

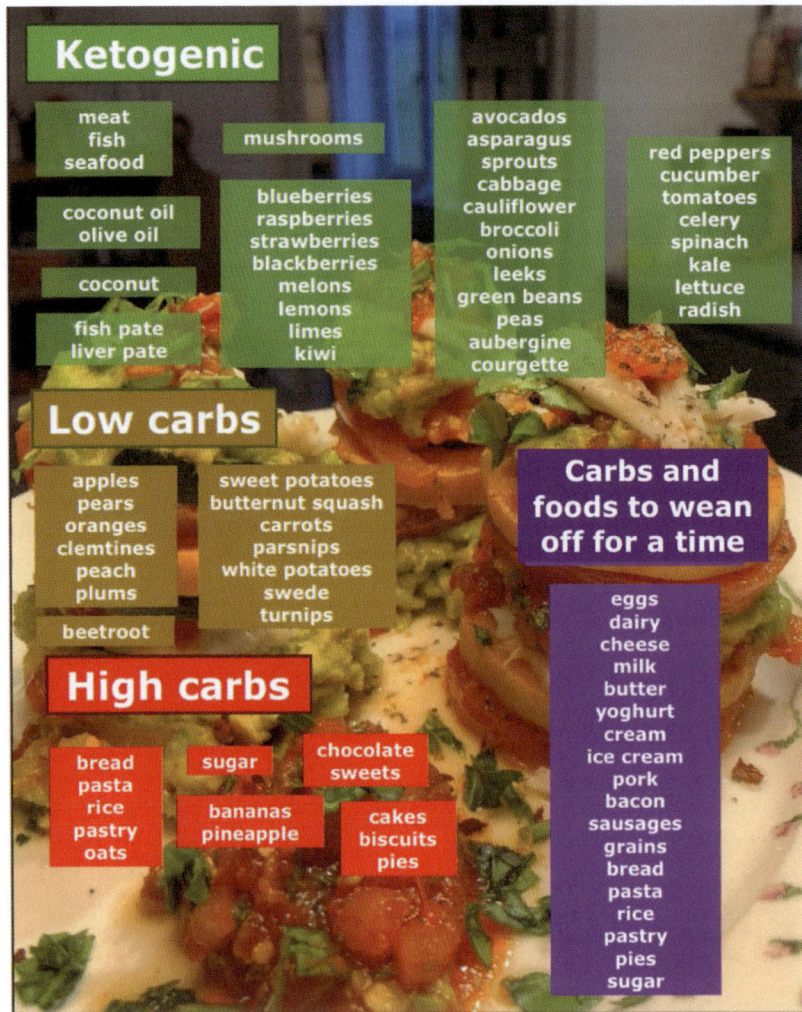

All about troublesome foods and drinks

Healing Chronic Illness: A Journey of Change and Transition

When we're chronically ill and suffering, the key to recovery lies in transforming our lifestyle. However, confusion often arises because there are so many diets and lifestyle choices—fasting, keto, carnivore, low carb, slimming clubs, and more. To complicate matters, foods often marketed as "healthy" can be problematic for those with chronic conditions. For individuals in good health, most foods might be fine, but for those struggling with illness, certain problematic foods consistently surface Dairy : Sugar : Eggs : Gluten and other grains (bread, pasta, oats, rice, pastry, etc.) Pork products (high in saturated fats) Fizzy drinks and squashes. Alcohol, vinegar, and fermented foods (e.g., kefir) Legumes and nightshades for some (e.g., tomatoes, peppers, eggplants)

Where to Begin?

On a healing journey, it's best to start by eliminating the most obvious culprits—dairy, sugar, and gluten. For those with autoimmune diseases, going completely grain-free is often necessary. Gluten reactions can persist for up to three months, and in sensitive individuals, the body may react to all grains as a threat due to gut inflammation and permeability (leaky gut).

To heal the gut, grains should be replaced with root vegetables like sweet potatoes, butternut squash, carrots, and parsnips. These are easier to digest and less likely to cause inflammation.

Hidden Threats in Everyday Foods
Refined sugar is pervasive in supermarket products—from sauces and ready meals to seemingly innocent items like mint sauce. Dairy, too, poses challenges: it's high in fat, often contains hidden sugars, and lacks Fiber. While marketing campaigns have tried to position dairy as healthy by highlighting added probiotics and fruit, these additions often mask its inherent drawbacks. Fermented foods like kefir may seem beneficial, but there are simpler, gentler ways to support gut health. Probiotic-rich options like bananas and onions often work better for sensitive individuals. Breaking Down Food Myths. Dairy: Stimulates dopamine, creating cravings much like sugar. Salt-laden cheese acts as a stimulant for the adrenals. Eggs: High in cholesterol and fat but devoid of fibre. They can constipate and burden the liver, especially in those with compromised digestion. Vinegar: Harsh on teeth and the liver. Alternatives like lemon or ginger water offer far more benefits. Nuts and Seeds: Often difficult to digest. Almonds with husks, for instance, contain anti-nutrients that need removal through soaking. Beware of nut butters with added oils, which can make them inflammatory.

The Hardest but Most Effective Change
Adding new, healthy foods to your diet is easy, but the real challenge lies in what you can remove. This process requires patience and a willingness to find replacements that bring joy and satisfaction. For example, coffee—a staple for many—can disrupt the gut microbiome and overstimulate the adrenals, leading to cortisol surges, stress, and anxiety. While supplements can help, there's no substitute for transitioning to a nourishing diet that supports gut healing and, in turn, improves chronic health conditions.

Planning for Success
Healing isn't just about food—it's also about navigating social situations and daily life. Dining out or attending events requires preparation to ensure safe, enjoyable choices. Over time, these adjustments become second nature, and the rewards—improved health, clarity, and energy—are well worth the effort. This journey is about reclaiming your well-being and rediscovering the vibrant life that chronic illness may have overshadowed. It takes time, but each small, consistent step brings you closer to healing.

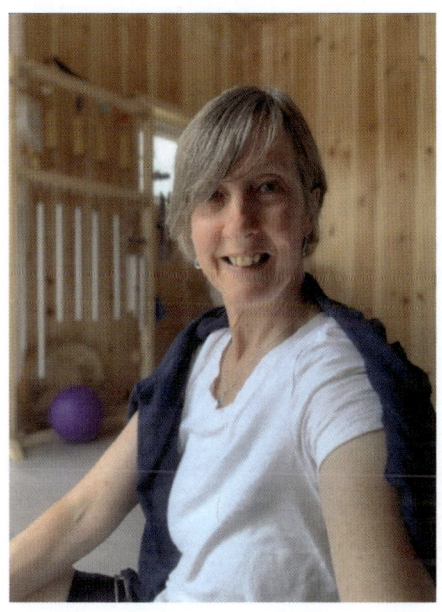

Juicers and Blenders: Essential Tools for Healing

Two indispensable kitchen tools that can accelerate healing are a good juicer and a reliable blender. These devices make it easier to incorporate nutrient-dense foods into your daily routine, providing vital support for recovery and overall health.

Juicers: Centrifugal vs. Cold-Pressed. There are two main types of juicers:

Centrifugal Juicers – These work quickly, using high-speed spinning blades to extract juice. They're convenient but can generate heat, which may reduce the nutrient content.

Cold-Pressed Juicers – Also known as masticating juicers, these use a slower, grinding process to extract juice, preserving more nutrients and enzymes. Though they take longer, they offer superior nutritional benefits. A juicer separates the pulp from the juice, leaving you with a concentrated liquid full of vitamins and minerals. The pulp can be composted or discarded. Juicing allows us to consume far more nutrients than we could by eating whole foods alone. For example, few people would eat an entire bag of carrots in one sitting, but juicing them makes it easy to drink their nutrients in just one glass.

Making Juices Palatable and Healing

On their own, certain vegetables like carrots may have a bland or unappealing taste. That's where good recipes come into play. Adding fresh herbs, roots like ginger and turmeric, and healing spices can transform your juice into a flavourful, medicinal drink. Fresh Herbs – Have antimicrobial properties that can help kill pathogens and parasites, detoxifying the body over time. Roots and Spices – Support gut health, enhance the microbiome, and act as powerful antioxidants. In today's toxin-laden environment, antioxidants are crucial for combating oxidative stress and promoting long-term health.

Blenders: The Smoothie Maker Advantage

Unlike juicers, blenders retain the pulp and Fiber, blending all the ingredients into a smoothie. This means you're consuming the whole food, which provides additional benefits like Fiber for digestive health. Smoothies are versatile and can include a variety of ingredients like fruits, vegetables, nuts, seeds, and superfoods. They're perfect for a quick meal replacement or a nutrient-packed snack.

Cold pressed juicer   **centrifugal juicer**

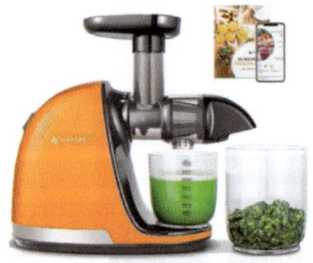
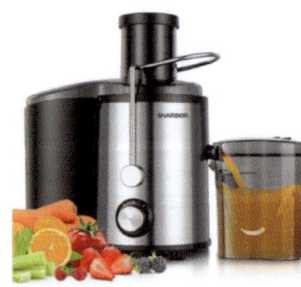

Nutri bullet blender....smoothie maker

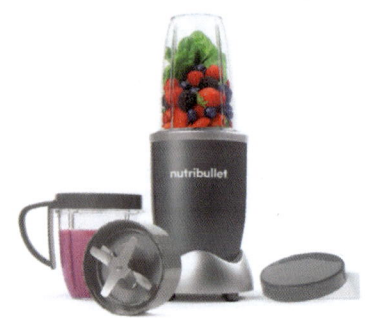

Breakfasts, juices, smoothies and herbal teas etc

How we start the day is most important, we may need to change from grabbing a coffee and putting the toaster on. Our livers like to cleanse in the morning and what we choose can aid this process. The first drink of the day can be A herbal tea, or a lemon water or a ginger water is best. In summer cold drinks are fine, but maybe in winter like me, you may wish a warm drink. Don't poor a boiling kettle onto lemons, as the water needs to be cooled, or it harms the effects of the lemon.
Drinks to wean off from would be fizzy drinks, alcohol, squashes, bought fruit juices etc.

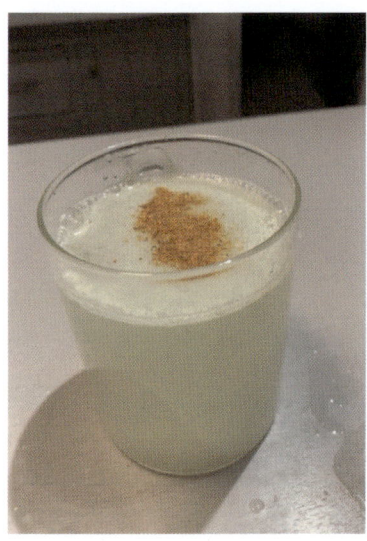
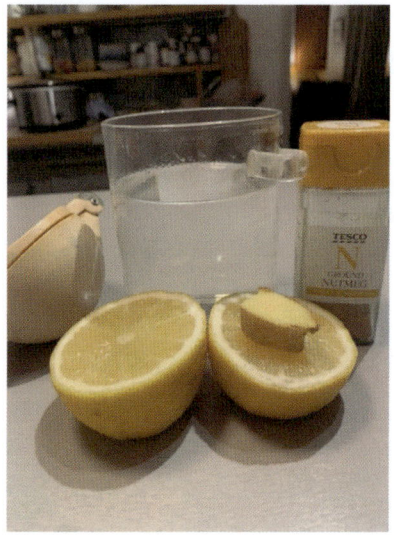
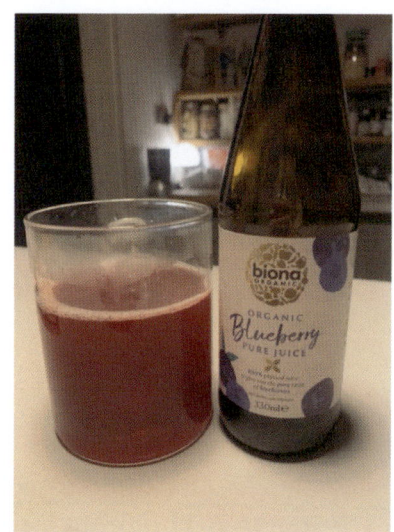

Lemon and ginger warm tea with added spices or either nutmeg or cinnamon is a good choice. Lemons are a powerful healing fruit that contain phenomenal antibiotic and antiseptic qualities. They cleanse the digestion and liver and hydrate, even though they are an acidic fruit they have an alkalinising effect on our bodies and cells. Lemons are also rich in bioflavonoids which can significantly boost the immune system and reduce inflammation in the body. Lemon juice is known to be particularly beneficial for colds, coughs and sore throats etc.
Try to find herbal teas like these, camomile, hibiscus, lemon balm and thyme etc, or just make up some mixtures of our own.

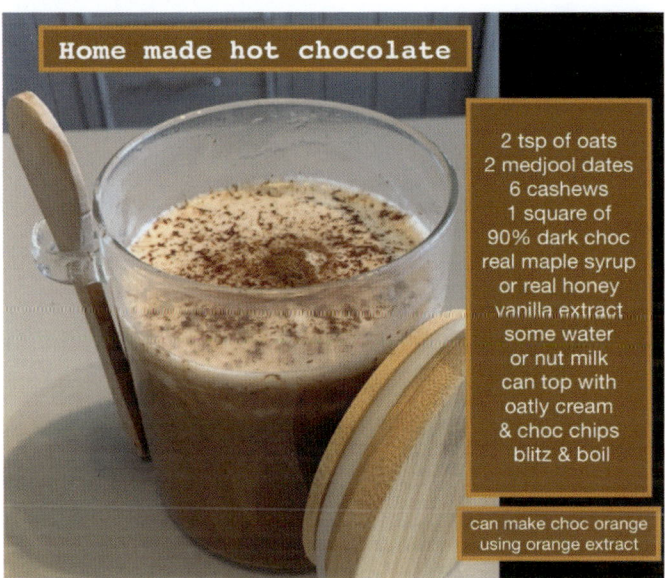
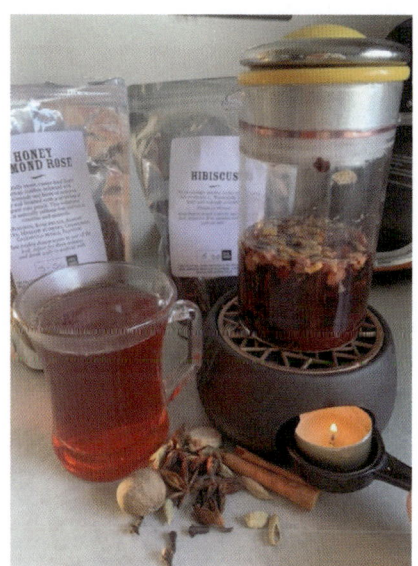

Harms of coffee [pubmed.com]
The Effects of Coffee on Health

- **Blood Flow and Oxygen:**
  Coffee slows blood flow to the brain by 22-30%, reducing oxygen delivery to cells.
- **Bone Health:**
  - Coffee consumption can reduce bone density, increase fracture risk, and lead to bone loss.
  - Higher caffeine intake has been associated with lower levels of magnesium and vitamin D, both essential for bone health.
- **Stress and Anxiety:**
  - Coffee raises cortisol levels (the stress hormone), contributing to stress and anxiety.
  - It acts as a psychoactive stimulant, speeding up heart rate, blood pressure, and thought processes, which can worsen anxiety and mental health issues such as bipolar disorder and depression.
- **Dehydration and Nutrient Loss:**
  - Coffee is a diuretic, leading to fluid loss and potential dehydration.
  - It reduces the absorption of iron by 39% and depletes B vitamins and magnesium.
  - Excess caffeine can cause electrolyte imbalances like hypokalaemia and hypophosphatemia.
- **Pregnancy and Brain Development:**
  Coffee consumption during pregnancy may negatively affect the baby's brain development.
- **Cholesterol and Heart Health:**
  Coffee raises cholesterol levels and may contribute to migraines.
- **Cognitive Health:**
  - Coffee decreases grey matter in the brain.
  - Studies link it to increased susceptibility to epilepsy.
- **Adrenal Function:**
  Chronic coffee consumption can lead to adrenal fatigue, causing low energy and high cortisol levels.
- **Histamines and Allergies:**
  Coffee increases histamine levels, which can aggravate allergy symptoms.
- **Vitamin and Mineral Depletion:**
  - **B Vitamins:** Coffee consumption reduces plasma levels of B vitamins like folate, riboflavin, and B6, even in healthy individuals.
  - **Vitamin D:** High caffeine intake has been linked to vitamin D deficiency.
- **Gastrointestinal Issues:**
  Coffee increases stomach acid secretion, which may lead to gastritis, ulcers, acid reflux (GERD), and other digestive problems.
- **PubMed Findings:**
  Research confirms coffee consumption depletes essential nutrients, including B vitamins, iron, and magnesium, especially with regular intake.

Caffeine works by antagonising adenosine receptors, which are found in the kidneys, brain, heart, and vessels. This increases glomerular filtration rate and inhibits sodium reabsorption in the renal proximal tubules + Coffee can have several negative health effects, including + Sleep disruption + Caffeine can block adenosine, a chemical that helps regulate sleep, leading to insomnia and difficulty sleeping + Anxiety + Caffeine can make anxiety symptoms worse because it stimulates the nervous system + High blood pressure + Coffee can be dangerous for people with high blood pressure because it stimulates the nervous system + Digestive issues + Coffee can increase stomach acid secretion, which can lead to poor digestion, nausea, heartburn, and other digestive issues + Rapid heart rate + Caffeine can cause your heart to beat faster and may lead to an altered heartbeat rhythm + Addiction Caffeine can create a physical dependence and chemical changes in the brain, leading to addiction + Dehydration + Caffeine can lead to dehydration, which can be dangerous for your health, especially if you have heart disease + cardiovascular disease + Long-term heavy coffee consumption may increase the risk of cardiovascular disease.

These are healthier alternatives to conventional coffee.

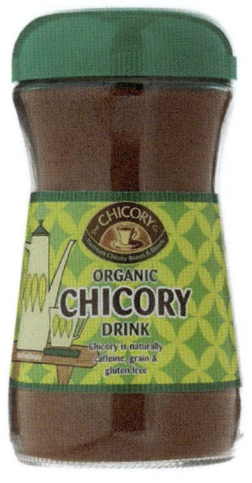 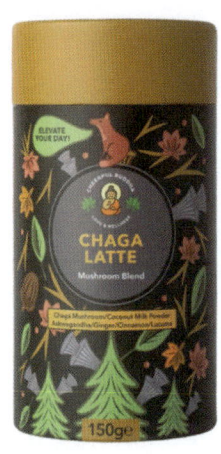 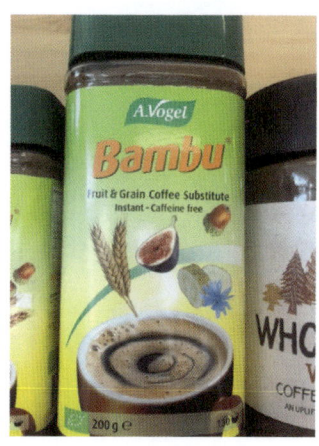

There are many healthier choices than coffee and the usual black tea. As these both slow down nutrient absorption. Changing habits can take time, but when we are chronically ill, it's all helping us heal. Caffeine is an adrenal stimulant which over times exhausts the adrenal glands.
Lynn's homemade hot chocolate = add one medjool date to a blender + a tsp of GF oats [or 2] + a dash of vanilla extract or orange extract + one square of dark chocolate [85%] [or orange choc] + one tsp of ground almonds [or a few cashews, or you can leave the nuts out if not wanted] + small cup of water = blitz and add to a pan and simmer and serve and enjoy. [can add cinnamon, nutmeg, ginger, if wished for]   The cream here is a dairy free one and it was Christmas.

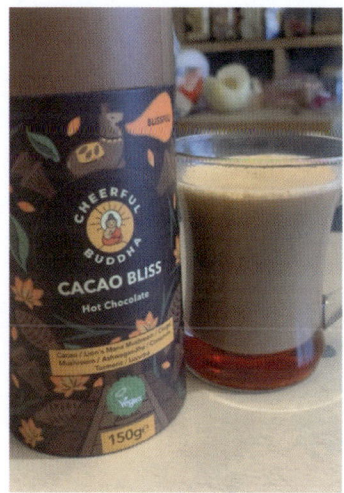 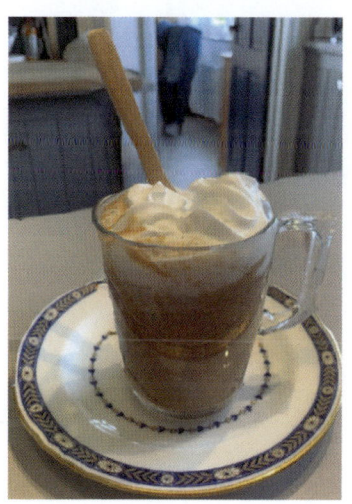

Juicing

Juicing is a great way to get more hydration and nutrition into our body. It's helpful also for people for whatever reason can't eat very well. Some people do juice fasts, others just have one juice a day. Celery is the top healing juice, its best to have alone and to start off with a small cup for a few days before building up to a pint or more after a week or so. If the celery is fresh and kept in the fridge it tastes nice. When it is going brown in colour after juicing, it doesn't taste so nice. If you don't like celery then there are many more to choose from. First thing mornings is the best way to start juicing and it takes time to get used to the habit.

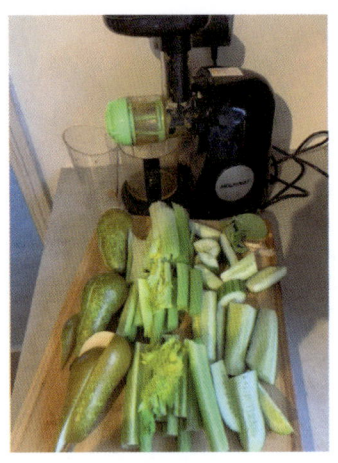
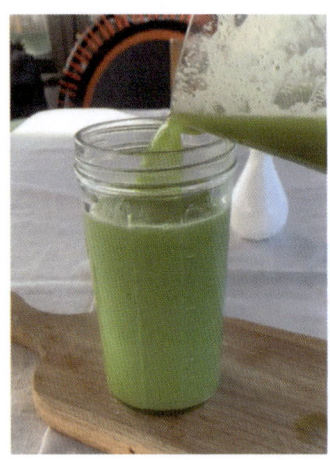
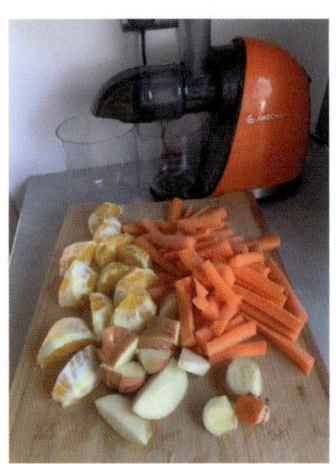

Adding fresh herbs like coriander, basil, flat leafed parsley, mint and using fresh herbs like ginger and turmeric. This make the juices super healing in their abilities to claw out heavy metals and killing off parasites and pathogens etc. These pictures will give you an idea of recipes to use. Also, you can look up some on the internet or buy a book. Start off with a small juice and as your body gets used to them, you can have more. In summer they are easier to consume, but I juice throughout the winter too. With juicing we don't consume the pulp, just the liquid juice. Juicing at the start of the day keeps us super hydrated. Also, we may not need a breakfast until later in the morning.

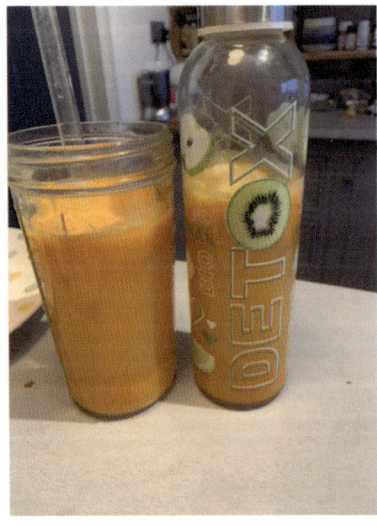
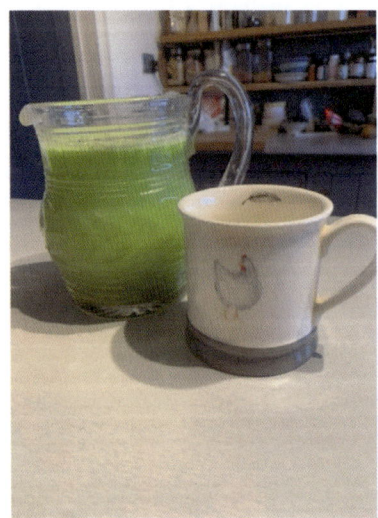
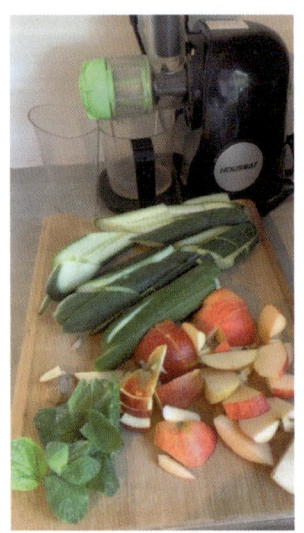

Colour is important with a smoothie and getting the taste right, we can add a little real honey or real maple syrup if desired. [don't have beetroot everyday as it can be in high doses toxic to the liver, if the wee turns red, then stop having it, is a good maxim]

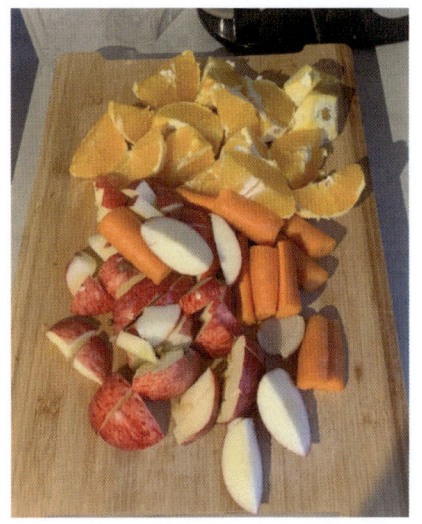
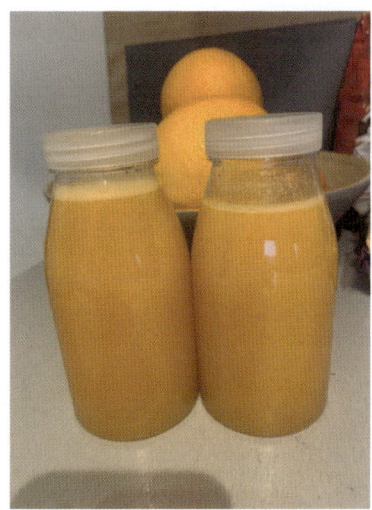
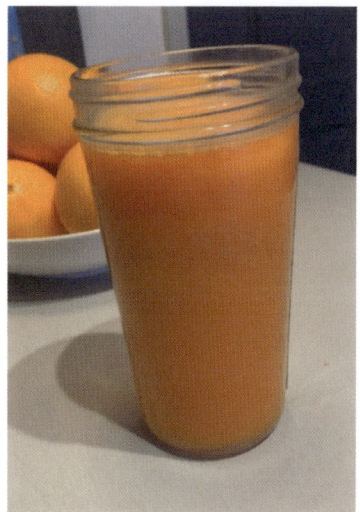

Juice is best fresh and consumed in a few hours, but it can be packed up and taken with us.
There are many juices to try, if you search online or buy a book, adding spices, fresh herbs and roots like ginger and turmeric take them to the next level healing. Adding veg with the fruit instead of just fruit is best, especially if fruit is a worry because of high blood sugars. Start off with a simple recipe before trying out more complicated ones. As sometimes if we add too much they don't taste as good. Green juicing is especially helpful for cleansing the liver and kidneys. One of the greatest benefits of green juice is its ability to restore hydrochloric acid (HCL) levels in the body. Full of minerals that easily absorbed and also anti-inflammatory and anti-pathogens. These all help heal the gut microbiome.

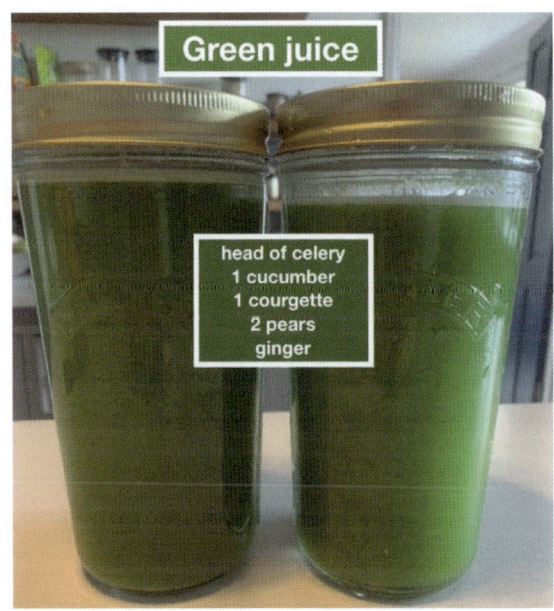
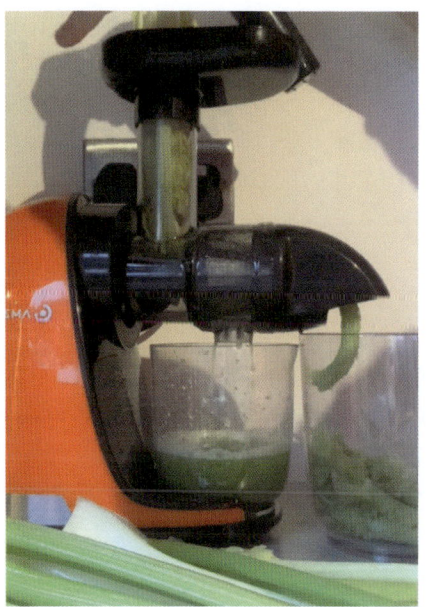

Smoothies

The top smoothie for healing is the heavy metal detox smoothie by Anthony Williams. It is a powerful healing smoothie we can have every day for a time or 3 times a week or when we wish.

Ingredients:
1 or 2 bananas
2 cups frozen or fresh wild blueberries, or 2 tablespoons pure wild blueberry powder, if you can't order this, have ordinary ones
1 cup tightly packed fresh coriander
1 teaspoon barley grass juice powder [this can be ordered on amazon as a powder with spirulina, Atlantic dulce all in all together]
1 teaspoon spirulina
1 tablespoon Atlantic dulce
1 or 2 fresh oranges, juiced
1 cup water, coconut water

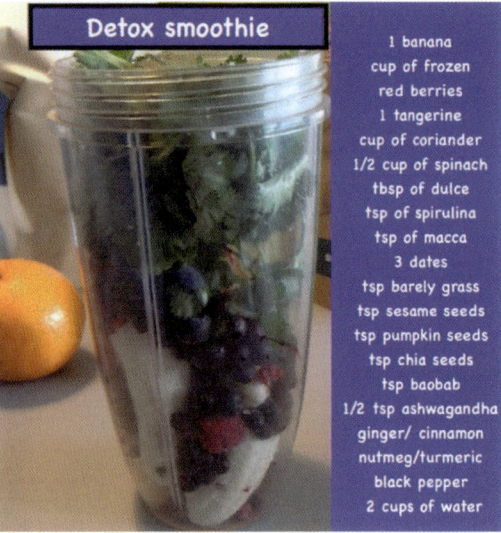
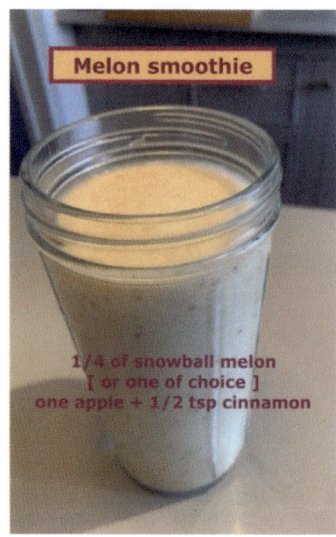
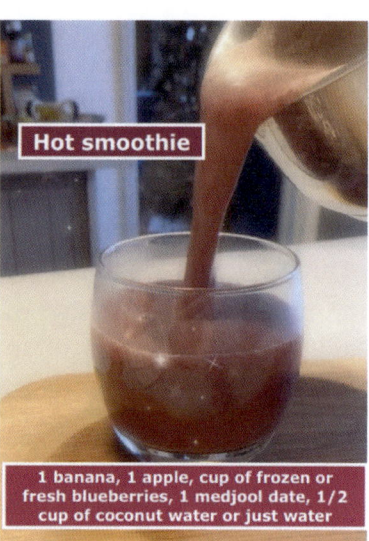

Red berries are super antioxidants and needed every day on a healing journey. Some people prefer a smoothie bowl, which can be made thicker and eaten with a spoon. The green smoothie we can, also add spirulina + barley grass juice powder. [to increase its healing abilities]

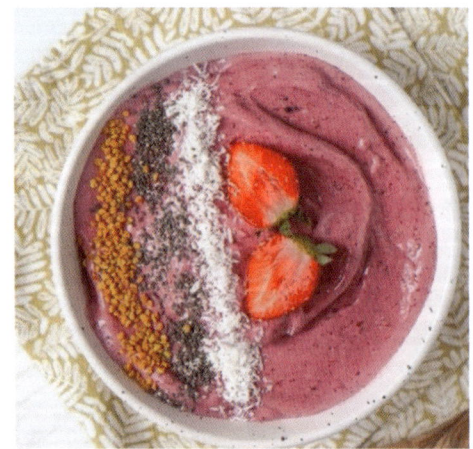
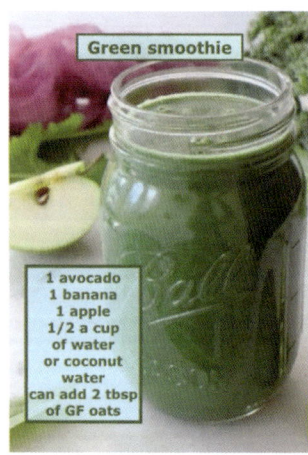

How to construct a great smoothie
1 First add the fruits, red berries are great antioxidants but not that sweet or fibrous, so I add either bananas or mangoes or oranges or pineapples to the smoothie,
2 add leafy greens, either spinach, which I like, or kale or an avocado,
3 some fresh herbs, either coriander, basil, flat leafed parsley, chives,
4 detox powders, like spirulina, barley grass juice powder, chaga mushroom powder,
5 coconut water or water [I avoid milks or nut milks]
6 can add nuts and seeds or nut betters or coconut oil [but for some these can be irritants]
7 spices and roots like nutmeg, cinnamon, ginger, turmeric,
8 some people like to add gluten free oats, which make for a filling meal, or they can be made lighter with just some melon and apple,

It takes time to invent one that suits you, either in a glass or even thicker in a bowl. If you like a little bit of real honey or real maples syrup can be added also. The trick is to NOT add to much water, as that dilutes the flavour, only add a little. If I make a melon or one with oranges, they really don't need any added water. Checking out some detox smoothies online or buying a book can be helpful.

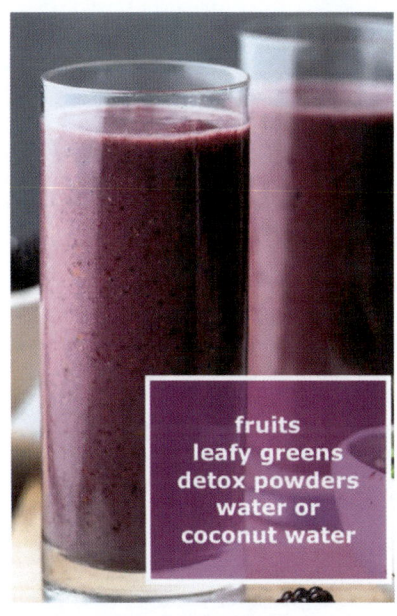

Recipe cold smoothie
Mug of frozen red berries of choice
or cherries
1 banana
1 apple or 1 pear
2 slices of pineapple
Cup of coconut water

Smoothies can be cold in summer and warm in winter. This hot banana one is, 1 banana, 1 medjool date, tsp of ground almonds, cup of water, dash of nutmeg, extra real honey if needed, then blitzed and warmed in a saucepan.

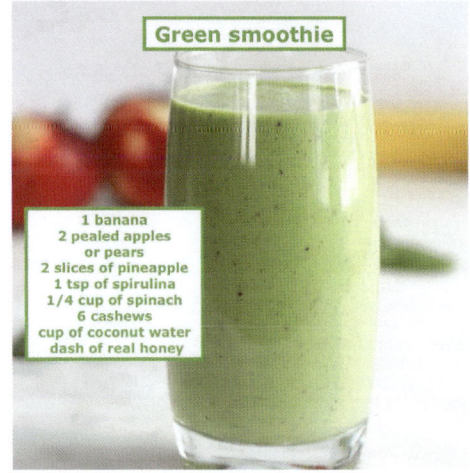

Green smoothie
1 banana
2 pealed apples
or pears
2 slices of pineapple
1 tsp of spirulina
1/4 cup of spinach
6 cashews
cup of coconut water
dash of real honey

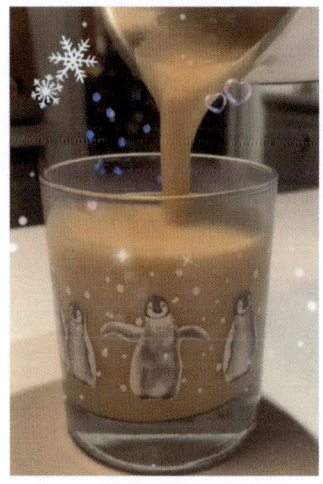

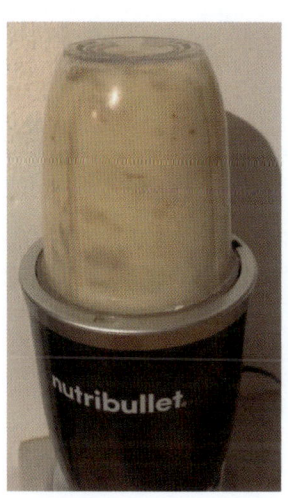

Fry up fruits and pancakes

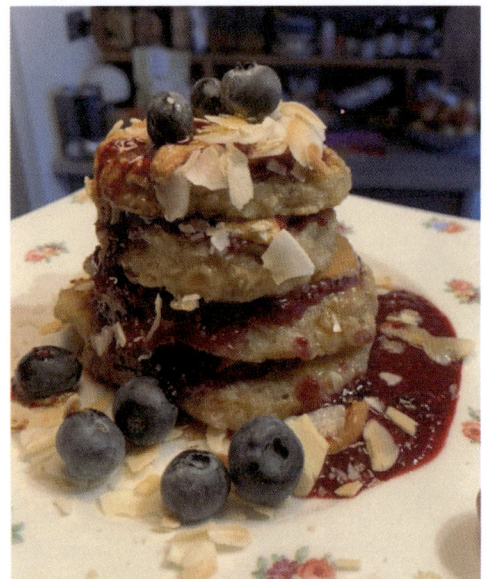

This is mashed banana with gluten free oats
A dash of water of nut milk. The jam is frozen red berries
With chia seeds and 2 tsp of real maple syrup.
I fried this is coconut oil on parchment in a frying pan to avoid sticking. I spooned 4 blobs onto the parchment paper. Then as I stacked them up, I added cashew butter and the jam in-between and then drizzled real maples syrup on top and added a few sliced bananas and coconut flakes.

These are fried fruits in coconut oil and a little real maples syrup or honey, and water, I didn't burn them and only gentle fried them. The apples are sprinkled with cinnamon, ginger and nutmeg, the bananas and mangoes o sprinkled with desiccated coconut. These breakfasts are better than cereals like muesli, granola and yoghurts, fruit is the best breakfast meal. I sometimes just have a juice and then later have something to eat. It all depends how hungry you feel first thing mornings.

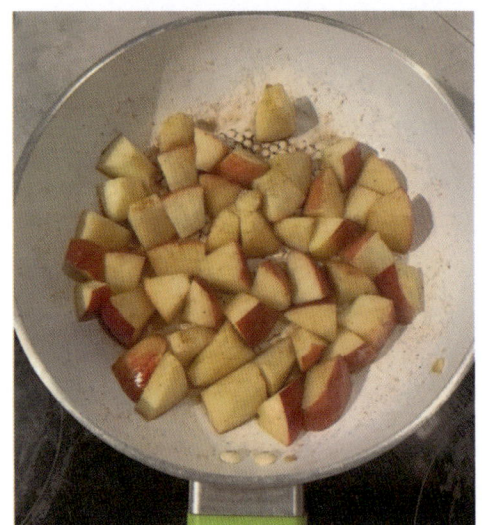

This one has is banana, GF rice Krispies, Oatley cream, cashew butter, medjool dates fried in coconut oil, maple syrup, coconut flakes and blueberries.

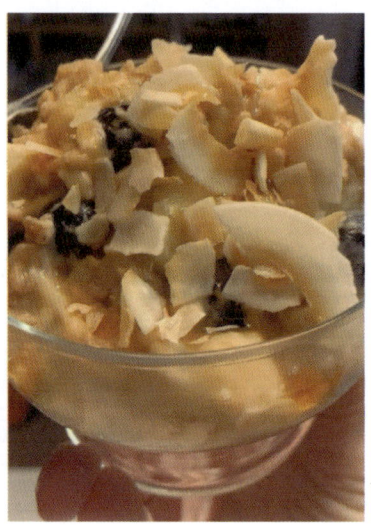
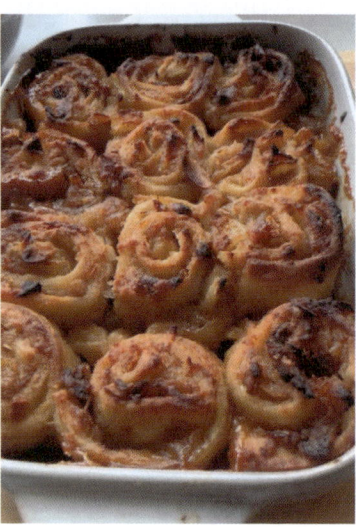
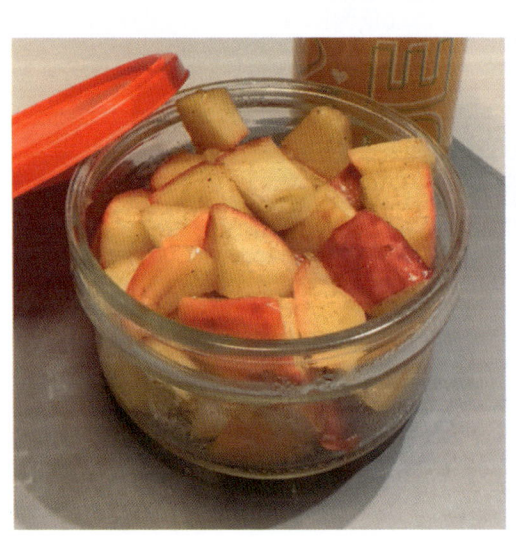

The swirl apple pie is Gluten free and sugar free, its fried apples in coconut oil, Medjool dates, cashew butter, maple syrup, flaked almonds, Oatley cream + water and we had a vegan ice cream on top. This was a special Christmas treat and not something I had 3 or 4 times a week.

Hot fried fruits in a caramel sauce. Sprinkled with soft coconut flakes or flaked almonds.

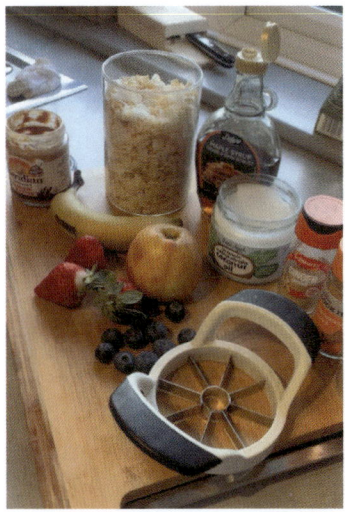 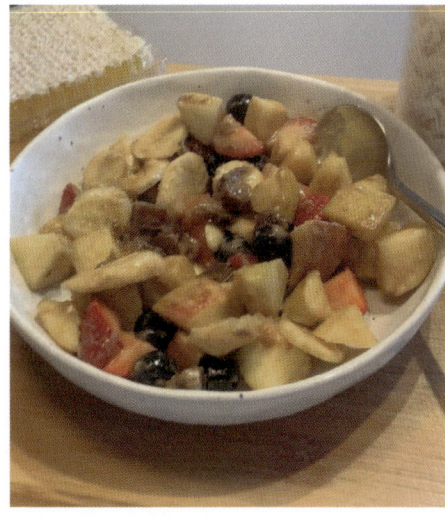

I add to a saucepan a tsp of coconut oil and an apple first, as it takes the longest to cook. Then I add a banana and some red berries, with cashew butter, medjool dates, then I add spices like nutmeg, cinnamon, ginger, just the tiny tip of a teaspoon of each. I then add a little water and either some real maple syrup or real honey. This is nice on a cold day. Hot fried fruit is a great breakfast. It's a lovely gooey mess.

Lunches and salads and soups
Many people are at work or out for lunch, so preparing things the night before and thinking about what you need to pack up. Lunch for many is a sandwich. I like to make a big salad with avocado and asparagus and sweet potato etc. Or a homemade soup to take to work. If I am home I have a cooked meal.

I slice sweet potatoes and place on a parchment sheet and pop them in the oven, no oil or fat is needed to cook them, and they cook in around 8 minutes, I flip them over half way through cooking. Meanwhile I prepare the salad to go with them. Which varies from mashed avocado with lemon [to stop them decolouring while I wait. Salmon or smoked salmon or cold turkey. I drizzle a little real honey on them after construction. All my recipes support the healing of the gut microbiome.

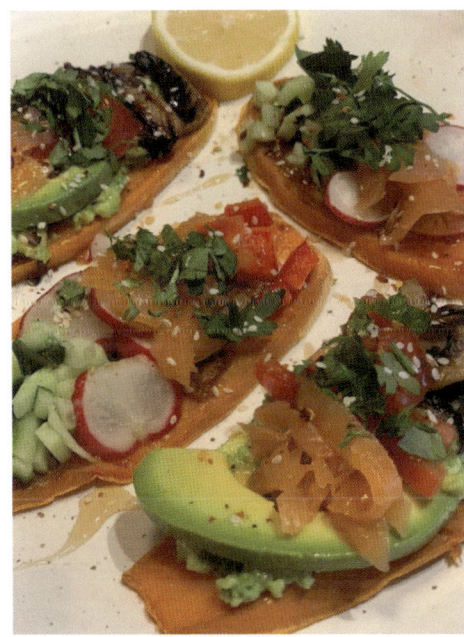 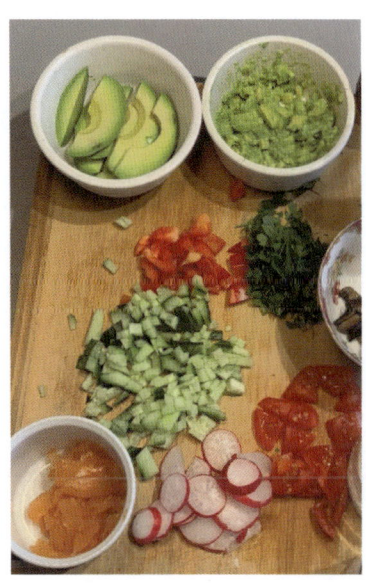 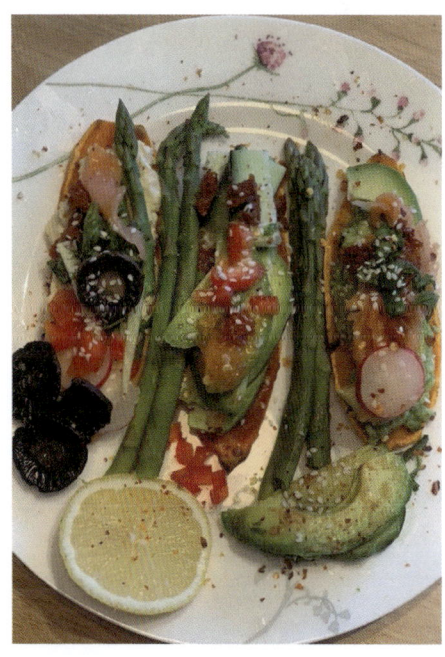

These are some lunches, a mixture between salad and cooked, depending on how cold and what time of year it is. I use as least amount of fat or oil I can, either coconut oil or olive oil.

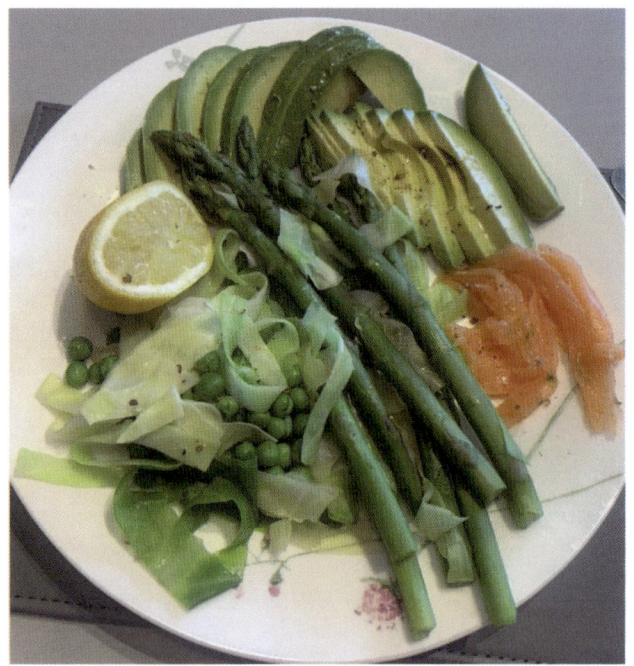
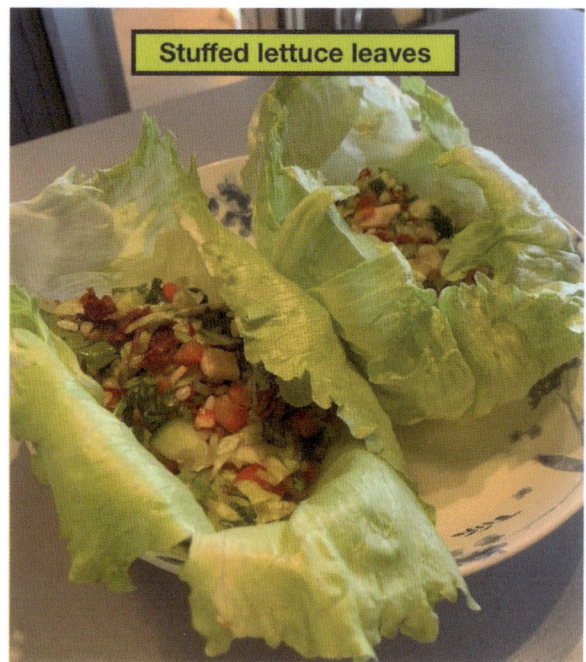

Greens are super healing foods and adding oily fish like salmon or sea bass, makes them super brain healthy meals. I use for a dressing a little real honey and some lemon, sometimes I make a garlic dressing with mustard and olive oil. Using fresh herbs like parsley, coriander or basil will make these meals even more medicinal. Stir fries are good as long as we don't buy the packet sauces, as they are full of sugar. Fruits and veg provide great fibre for healing the gut microbiome.

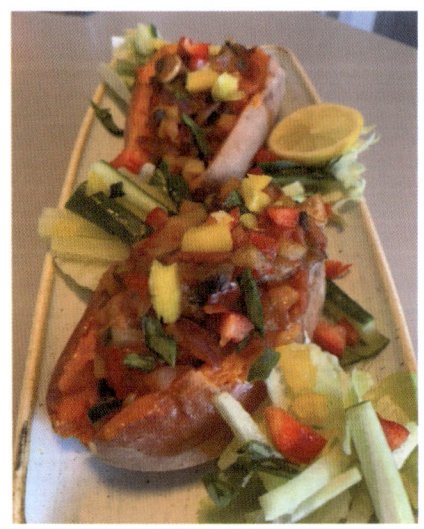
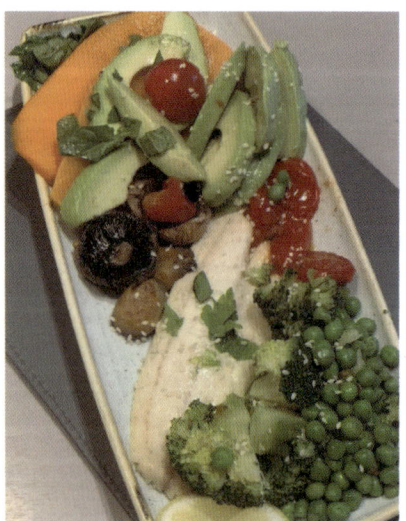
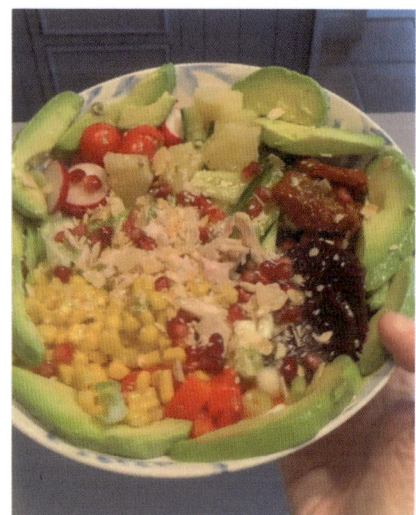

I don't eat bread now, so need the sweet potato for the carbohydrates. As salads without carbs don't fill us up long enough. This meal I used turkey bacon. Turkey is a tryptophan producing food, which is a precursor to serotonin, which makes this meal great for anyone with brain or mental health conditions. I fried them in a little coconut oil with a few sprouts.

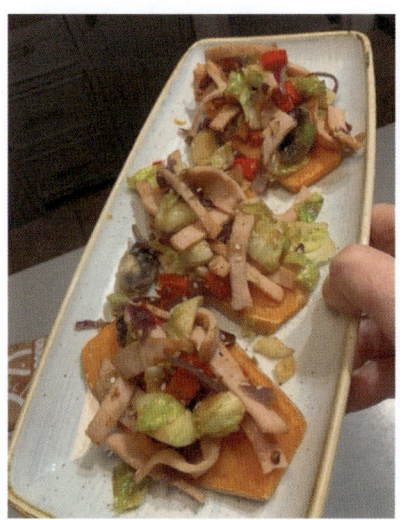 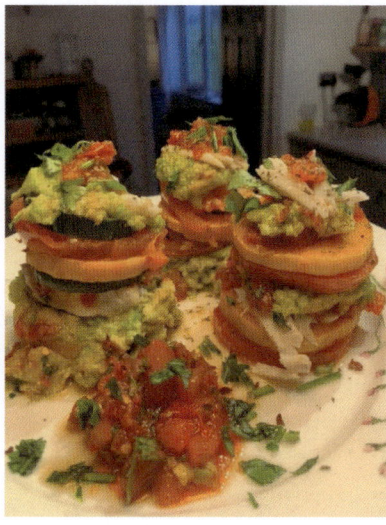 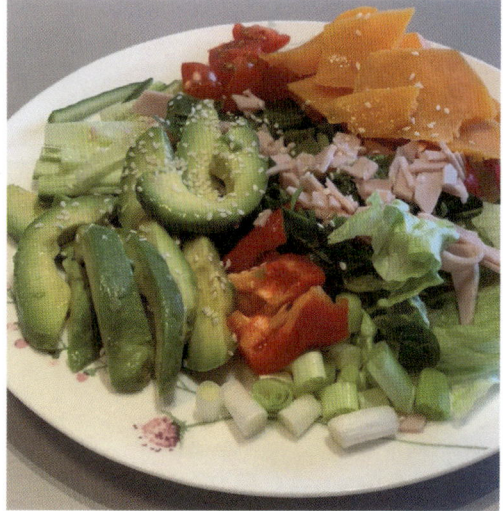

I sometimes mix cooked foods with salads, mostly I slice sweet potatoes and quickly pop in the oven, other times I steam them in a shallow frying pan with a little water. Unlike starchy white potatoes sweet potatoes cook a lot faster. Roasted they are lovely and have a nutty taste and are great for soups and stews and hot pots. The stackable's here are sea bass, and a spicy salsa, with basil.

Sometimes I like to cut up my salads tiny and eat with a spoon. I make my own dressing which are usually, real honey and lemon, sometimes garlic and mustard and a little olive oil. We don't need cider vinegar or fermented foods, or kefir to heal he gut microbiome, we need natural and raw meals.

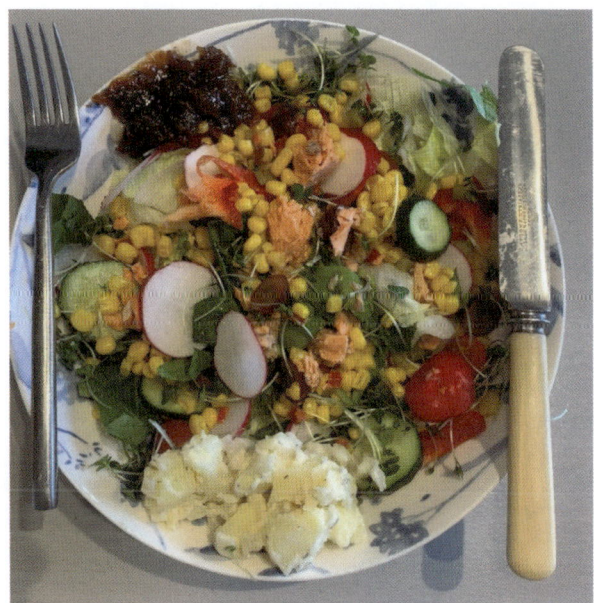 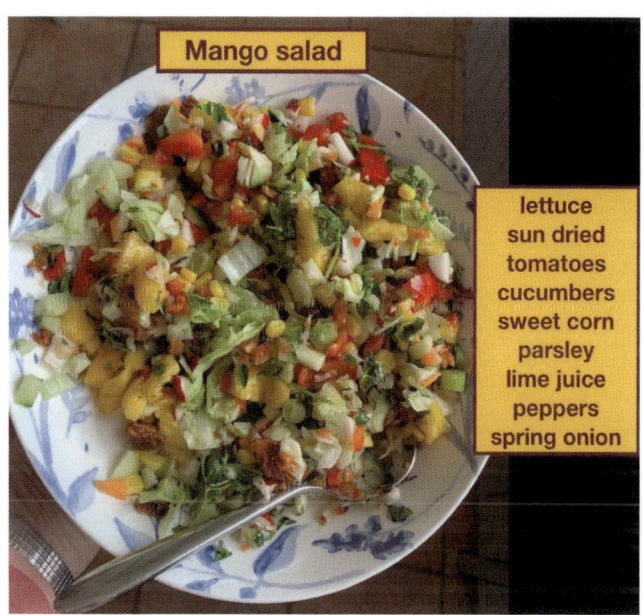

Mango salad

lettuce
sun dried tomatoes
cucumbers
sweet corn
parsley
lime juice
peppers
spring onion

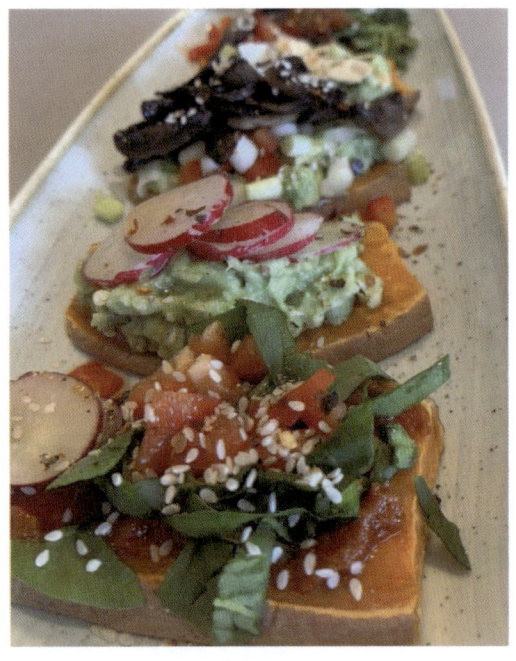
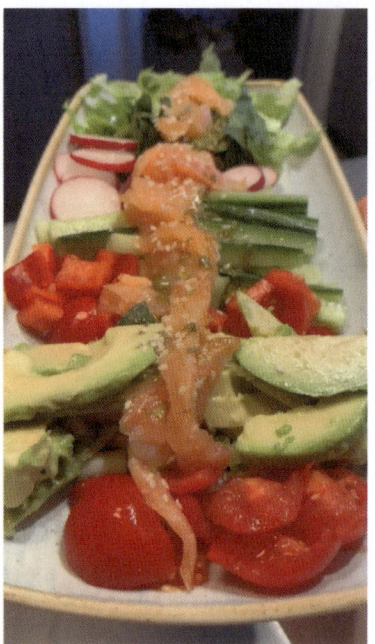

Spending time preparing and making a salad look nice is key to enjoying them. I like mushrooms, avocados, radishes, cucumber, spinach, but you may not like those and prefer other things. I don't really like kale, I prefer cabbage. I know kale is a super healthy leafy green, but I find it bitter and like spinach and cabbage better, so stick with what you like salad and greens wise. It's no good trying to eat things we don't like.

On a healing journey, it's important to have sweet things we enjoy and cooked things, meat and fish if we eat those. Some people are fine eating lots of beans and lentils, but for me they are not great things. I don't mind a few now and again, but I stick with salads items and veg, which I find easier to digest, as veg is living, where beans are more of what I call a suspended food item. A preserved food, like grains they are not grown into something. So, they are harder to digest for some of us. If you are ok with them, then fine, use them.

These are stacked sweet potatoes with
Filling of gluten free fish fingers and avocado.
[I rarely have frozen fish fingers, as mostly fresh]

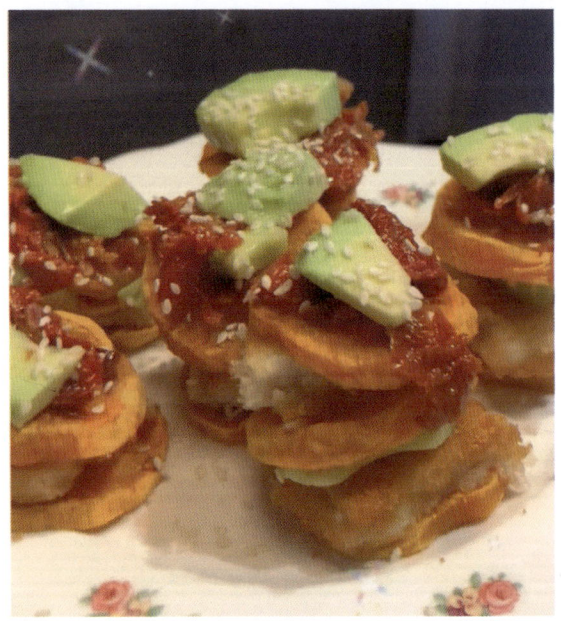

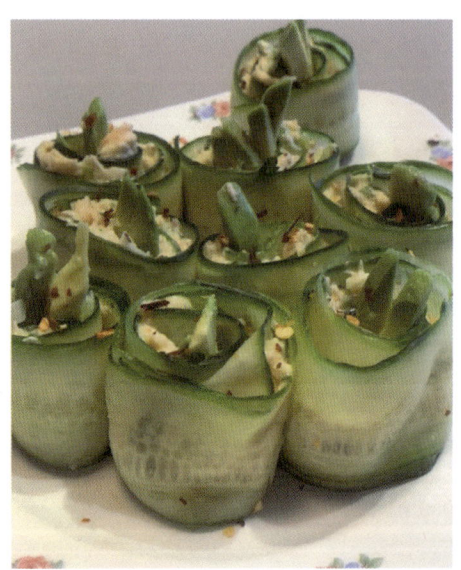

These stuffed cucumber rolls are filled with mashed salmon and a plant based cream cheese [as I avoid all dairy] I added a few slices of avocado. Chilli flakes and lemon, the lemon stops the avocado from browning.

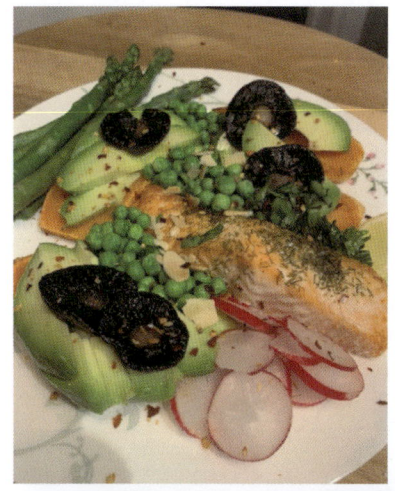

As you can see a lot of my lunch and salads have very similar things, as these are what I like. They are all anti-inflammatory and super healthy. I use a little coconut oil or a little olive oil as I can. As I have enough fats when I have a meat dish.

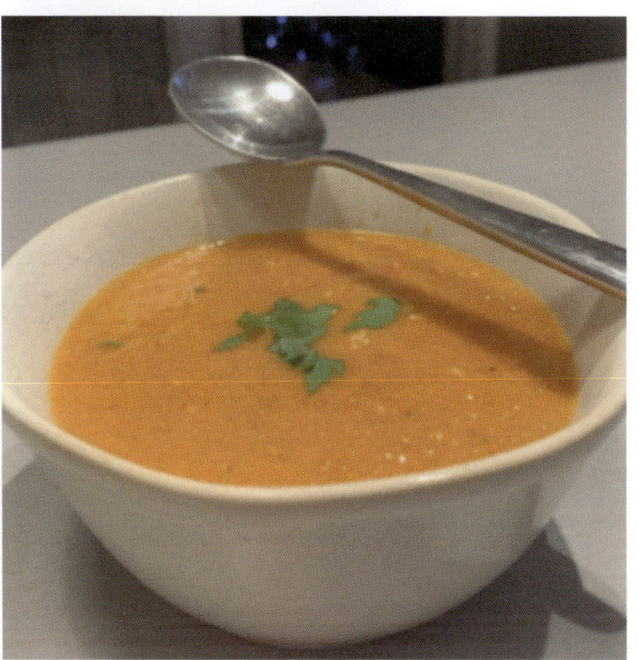

This is one of my favourite soups to make. I line a tray with parchment paper and cut up butternut squash, sweet potatoes, onions, red peppers, carrots, lots of garlic, tomatoes and fresh rosemary, sage, thyme and sometimes smoked paprika. I then sprinkle a little olive oil on and roast in the oven on the top shelf for 20 minutes or so. Then I take it out and add to a pan with a little water and a stock cube, some black pepper and a little pinch of Himalayan salt or sea salt. Sometimes it's not needed if the stock has salt in it. My daughter likes a little real honey with hers, when she makes it. Which is fine. This soup can be packed up for work and kept in the fridge for a few days. In autumn and winter, I have a lot of soups. They are super easy to digest meal and a much needed hot meal in cold weather.

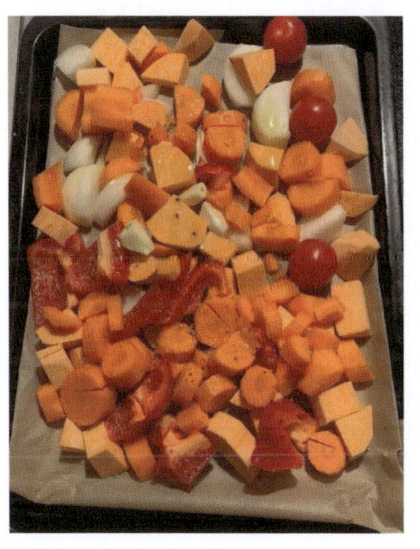 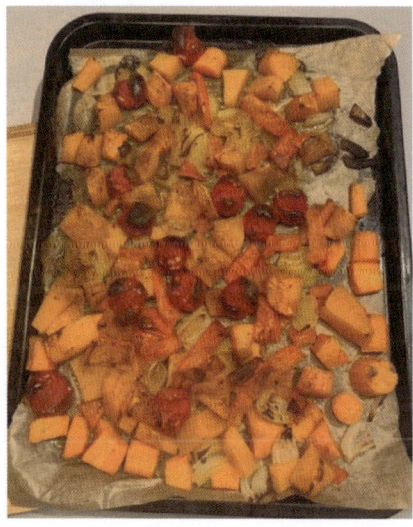 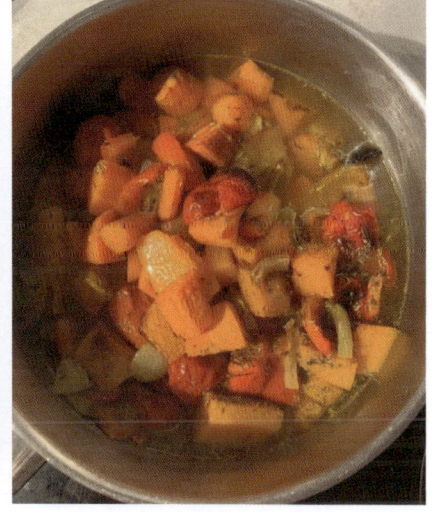

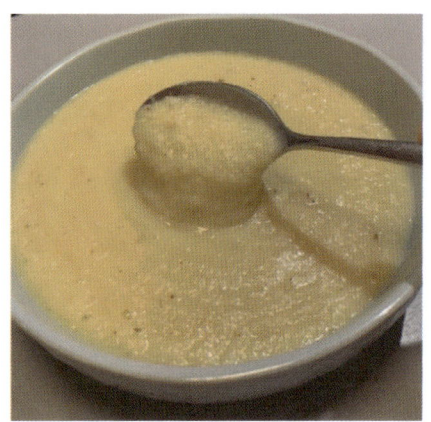

This parsnip soups is also another favourite of mine. It's very similar process to the last soup, in that I add cut up parsnips, onions and herbs to a parchment lined tray and roast in the. Then I add to a pan with a little water and vegetable stock cube. And blend with a hand blender until smooth. Roasting the parsnips makes them taste so much nicer than just boiling them, we can also add a little real honey. Soup is a good meal for gut health.

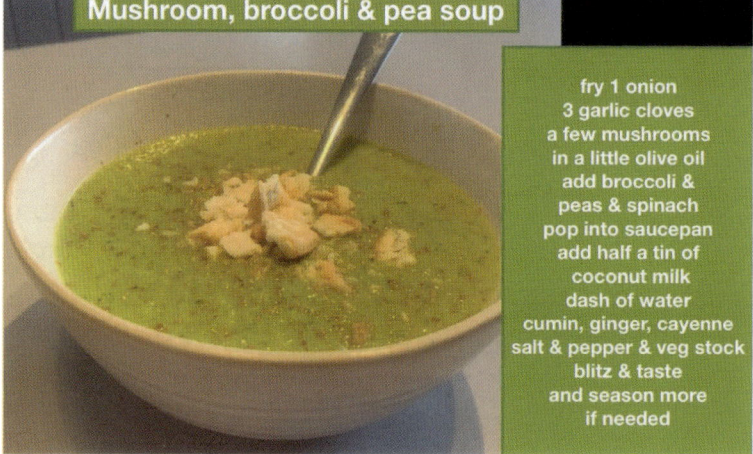

Mushroom, broccoli & pea soup

fry 1 onion
3 garlic cloves
a few mushrooms
in a little olive oil
add broccoli &
peas & spinach
pop into saucepan
add half a tin of
coconut milk
dash of water
cumin, ginger, cayenne
salt & pepper & veg stock
blitz & taste
and season more
if needed

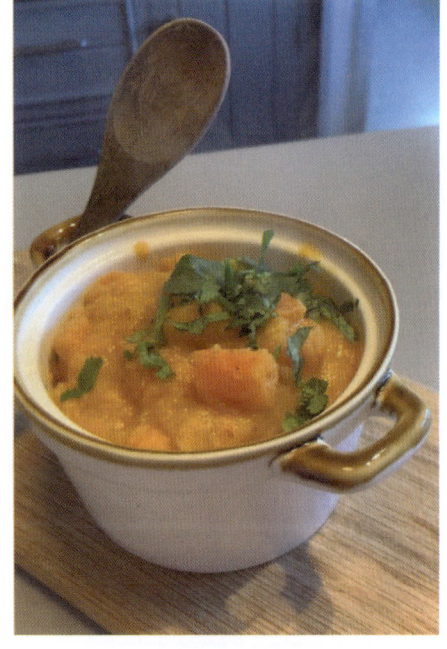

This little pot soup, was a tray bake of root veg, butternut, carrot, sweet pots, red peppers, garlic, ginger, turmeric, then added to a sauce pan with a tbsp of coconut cream, ½ a veg stock cube, cardamom, cumin, coriander, olive oil, hill salt and black pepper, some was blitzed, and some was left in cubes,

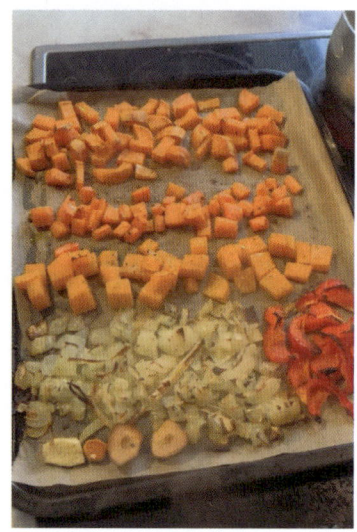

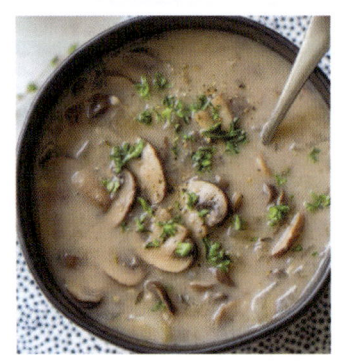

I also enjoy mushroom soup, but I don't have dairy cream, I just use a little coconut cream, also no added salt is needed as mushroom are salty enough. I fry them with onions and a little olive oil, making sure not to burn the oil, so only a gentle fry. Also, I don't have bread. A little gluten free toast or sough dough would be ok. But gluten is not good for any auto immune condition and some people will find that all grains will trigger inflammation.

Tea and traybakes and hot pots
I love a roast dinner and roast lamb, or chicken is my favourite. Sometimes we go out for a carvery, I avoid the Yorkshire puddings, stuffing, and sausages, as I don't eat pork. I always have lotas of veg with it and I don't have pudding straight away after, as puddings should be eaten away from the main meal. Our digestion likes to have different meals away from each other. The reason is down to bloating and digestion, it just makes it easier for our pancreas and gall bladder.

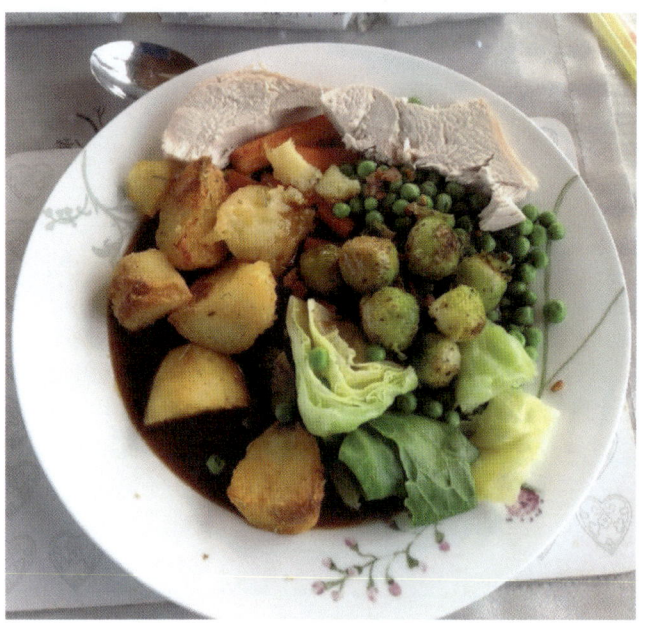
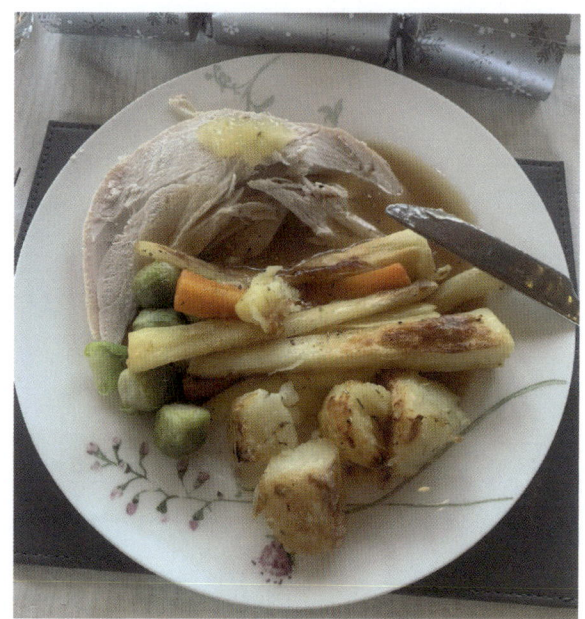

I love these sorts of meals and mostly cook them in a tray bake and add the gravy later. This kind of cooking means I can pop it on the middle shelf and leave it, as long as I add a little water and olive oil. Also, it saves washing up lots of pots and pans. I do cook the cabbage separately and add sprouts to a tray bake later on, as they don't need so much cooking. Practicing cutting the veg the right size for all the different cooking times takes a few goes. But I like this way of cooking.

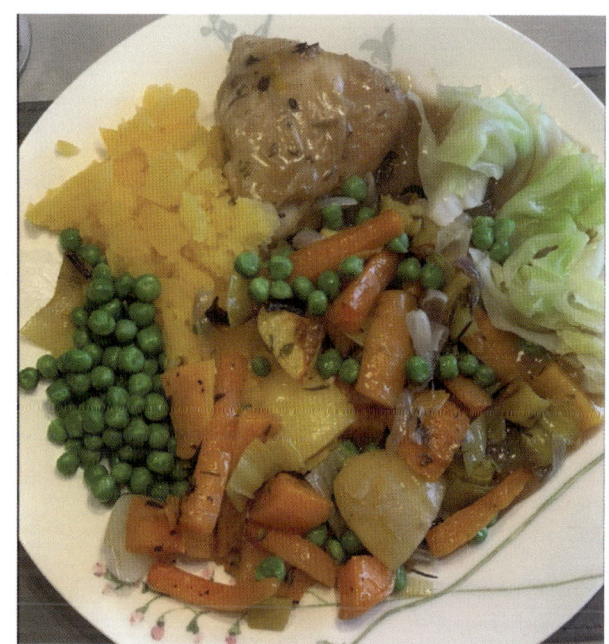

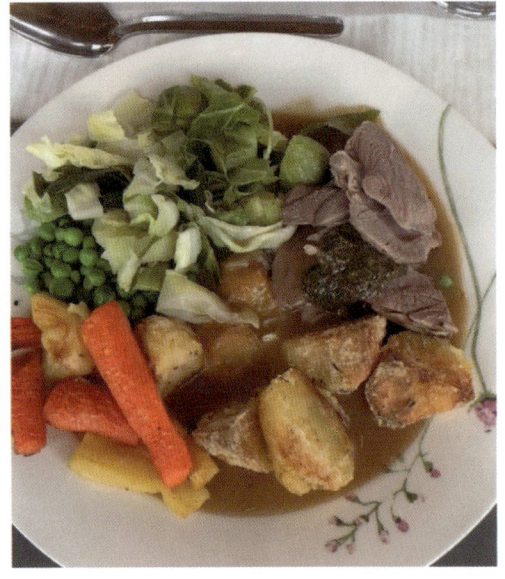

Roast dinners are fine if we have lots of veg with them and forgo the Yorkshire puddings. Having lots of greens and cooking them in a small amount of healthy fats like coconut oil of olive oil is best.

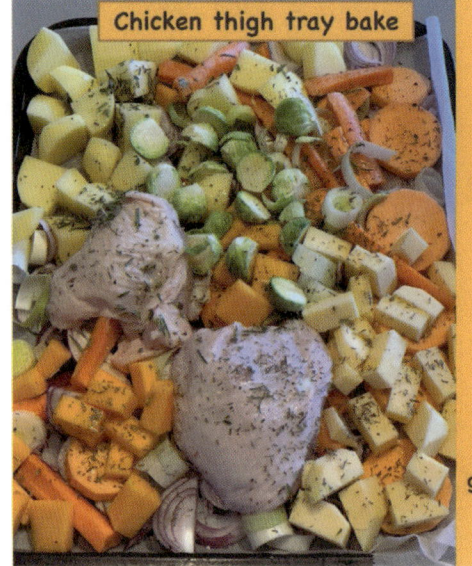

I have added the sprouts here, just to show you, but I didn't add them to the tray until most of the other things had been cooked. You can also cook them separately in a saucepan, it's up to you. Adding them at the start, overcooks them.
The gravy I use is Bisto powder with some plain gluten free flour.

Chicken thigh tray bake

2 red onions
leeks
carrots
sprouts
sweet potato
white potato
butternut squash
swede
fresh herbs
rosemary
sage
thyme
hill salt and
cracked pepper
olive oil

will make some gravy and pour on and do some cabbage & peas

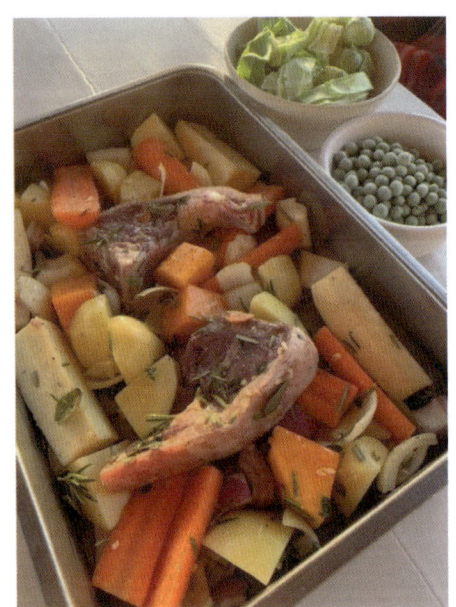

This is how I added everything to the tray with some water and olive oil, also, fresh herbs, which are all very healing. The peas and cabbage is separate.

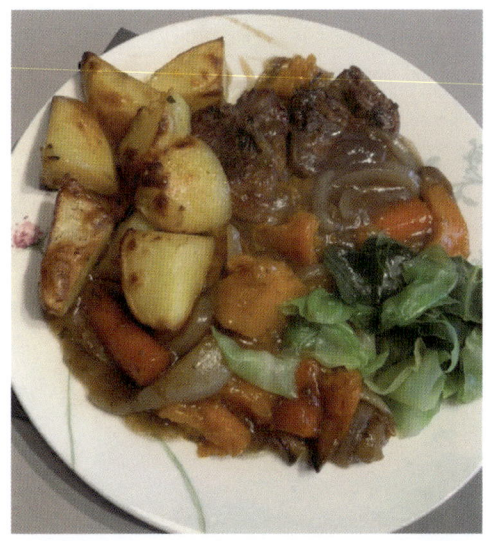

These meat and gravy meals I would only have two to three times a week and even less in the summer. I avoid pork and pork sausages and bacon. High fats are not good for digesting, or the gut microbiome.

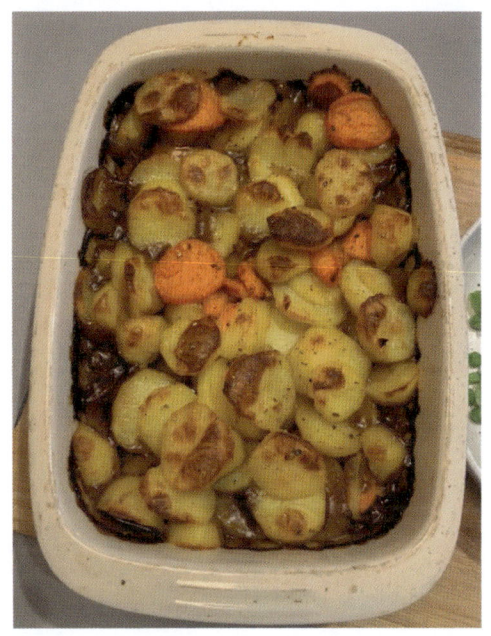

Cottage pie or shepherd's pie here is another, autumn winter meal. I tend to use sliced potato top and not mash, as that avoids butter and just a little olive oil is drizzled on top. I buy butchers mince and add onions, mushrooms and diced carrots and sometimes lentils to add to the veg content.

This meal was done in a hot pot and slowly cooked to bring the flavours out. With lots of veg added in like butternut squash and sweet potatoes. Then I also choose cabbage and peas to go with it, as greens are a much needed for food for health and healing.

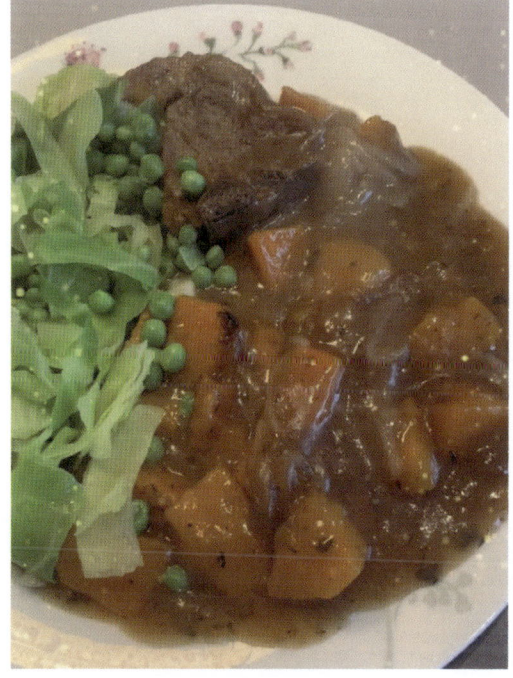

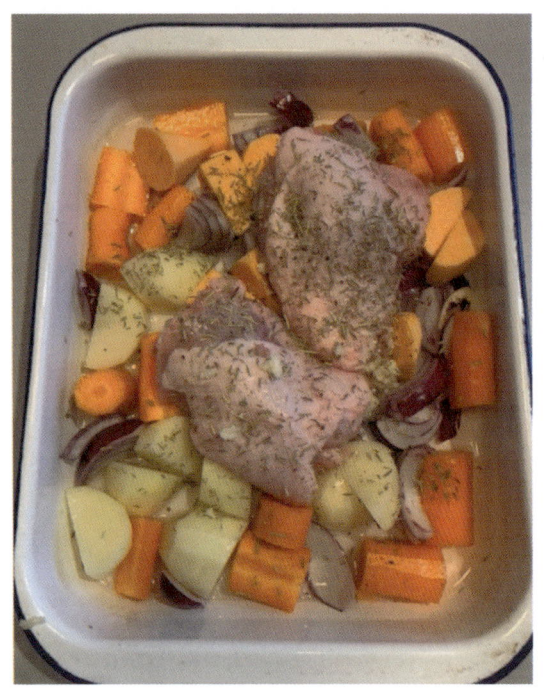

Another tray bake here using chicken thighs, sometimes I may make a gravy and other times I use a carton of tomatoes and add smoked paprika and harissa and a few medjool dates, which turns it into more of a Moroccan dish. I have white potatoes here as family was sharing this. I tend to stick with sweet potatoes. The fresh herbs are from my garden, they are important to have on any healing journey to add to juicers, smoothies and meals.

This is a chicken curry without, without the rice. This is a low carbohydrate meal which would be suitable for anyone with diabetes or anyone that wanted to lose weight. Sometimes we are not as hungry as other times and only need a lighter meal. Don't have the curry too hot if you suffer with inflammation issues.

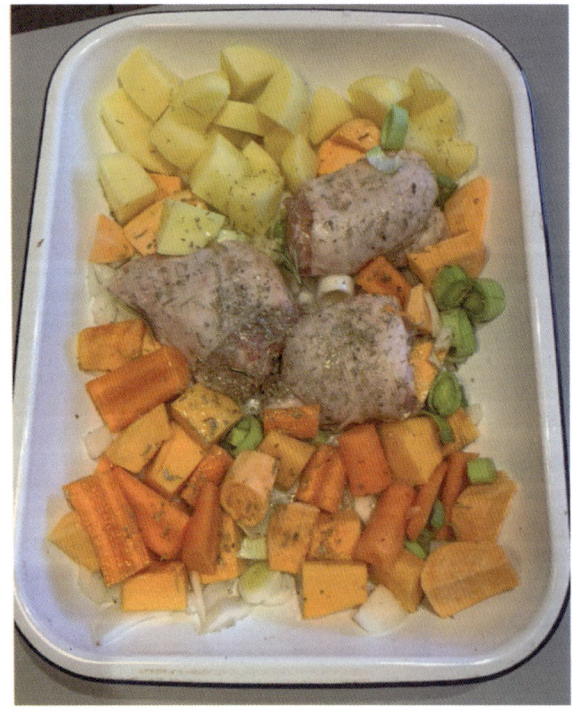
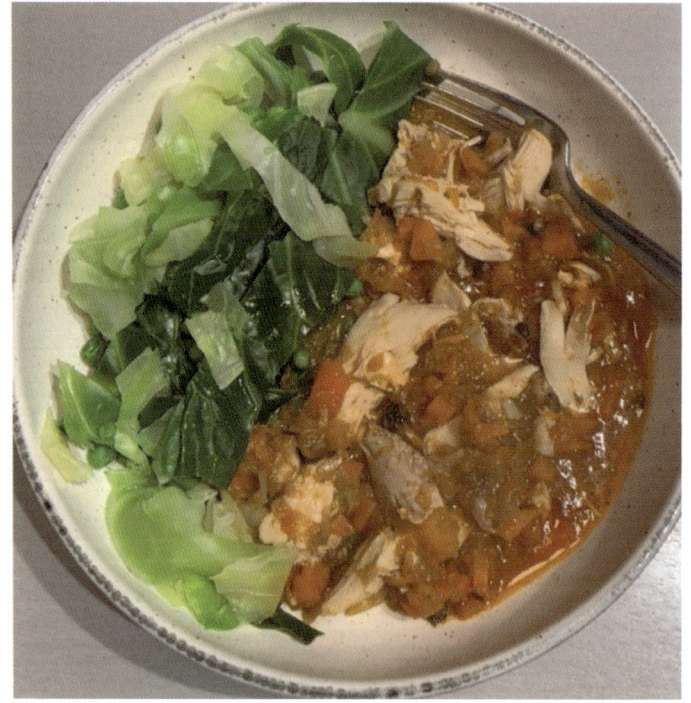

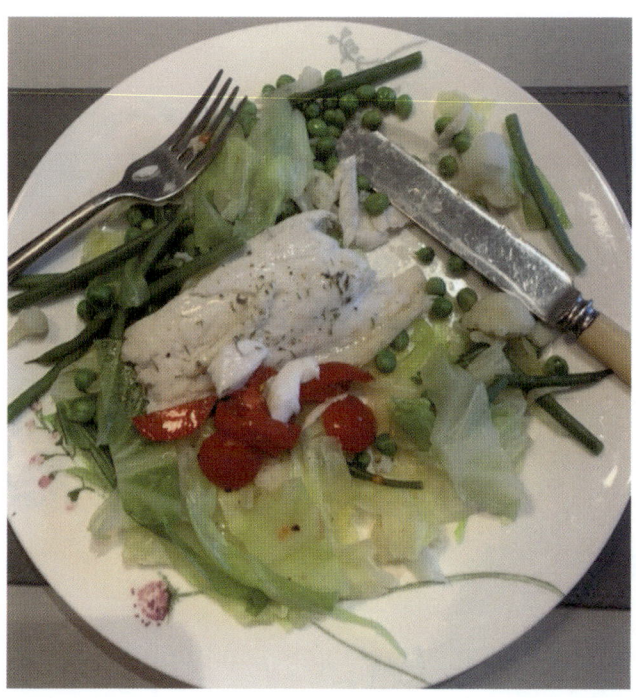 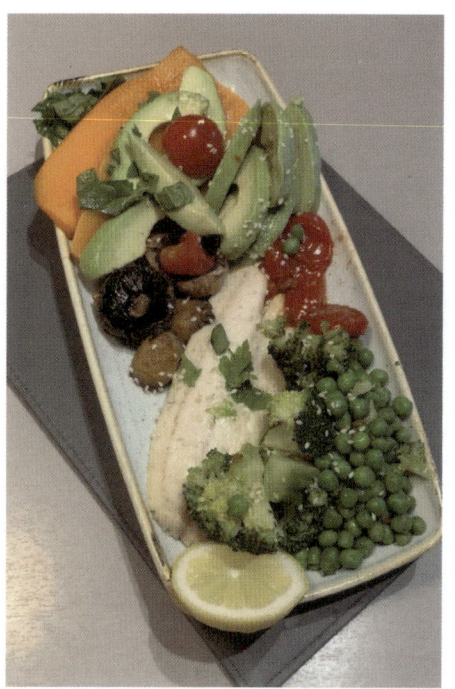

These two meals are lighter in carbohydrates and can be for lunch or an evening meal. Overground veg has less carbohydrates than underground veg. Not that over ground is better, it's just they have less glucose/carbohydrate in them, so we may need to eat more when we adopt a low carb diet. To avoid going hungry, as carbs fill us up and keep us fuelled for longer. Of course, these meals could be enjoyed at lunch or for dinner, depending on when you wish your main meal. It's best not to eat after 6 o'clock, as digestion slows down and going to bed on a full stomach is never a good idea. If you feel hungry evenings, then a healthy snack is fine. But try to have more earlier in the day and hydrate better to avoid this.

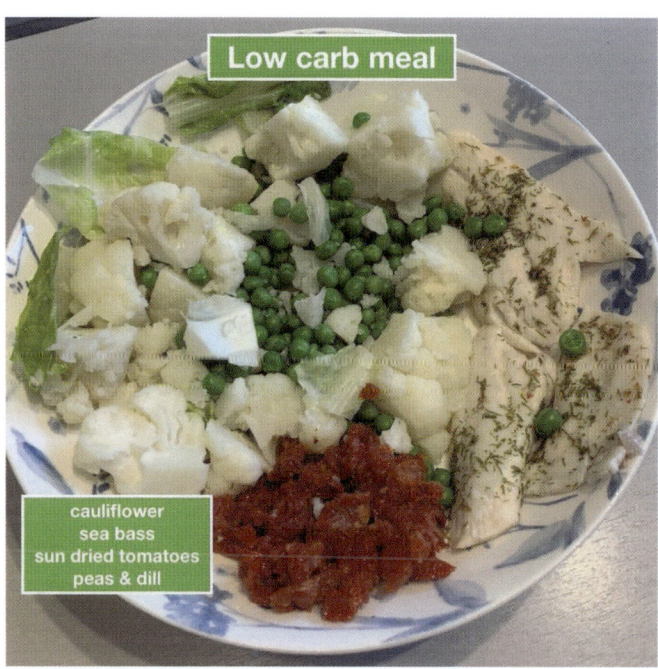 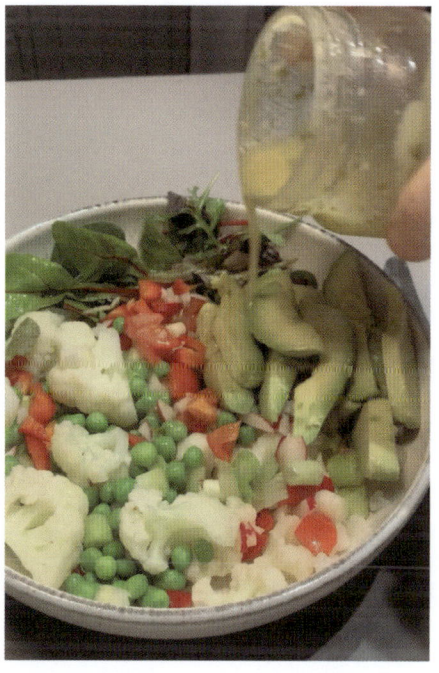

Low carb meal

cauliflower
sea bass
sun dried tomatoes
peas & dill

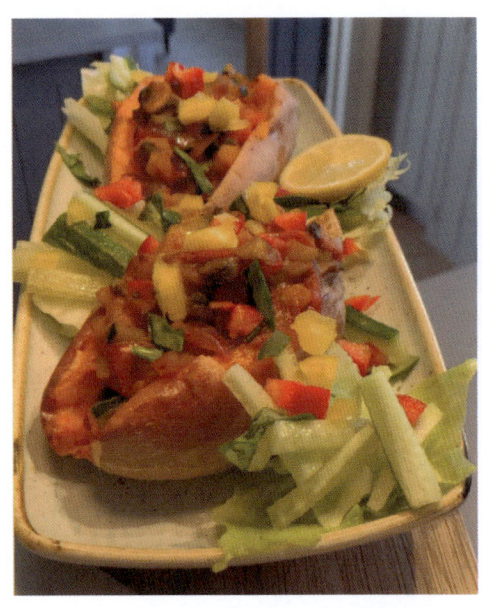 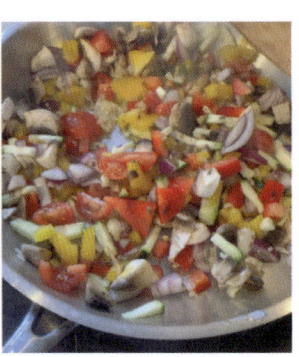 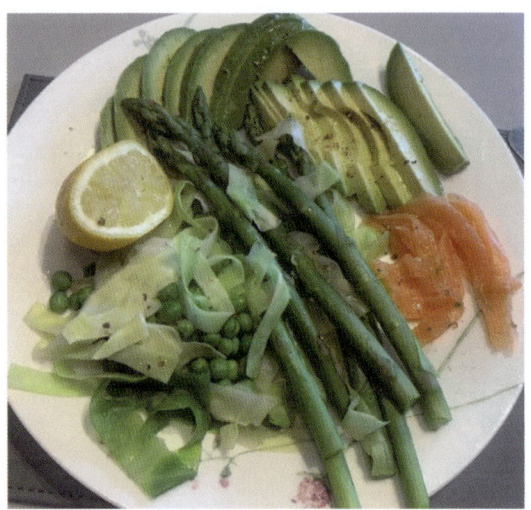

Sweet potatoes jackets here with a fried in coconut oil, mixed salad and veg in tomato sauce, with harissa, garlic, ginger, turmeric. The avocado and salmon salad is a meal of super healing greens, easy to digest and low in carbohydrates. When we're under stress, we tend to lose B vitamins more. Asparagus, is high in easily absorbable B vitamins, helps us reestablish our proper levels of these key nutrients. Avocados are a great brain food. A healthy source of omega-6 fatty acids, they can aid the central nervous system and are a good food for Alzheimer's, dementia, autism and mental health. Gut friendly meals here.

This is a hot and cold salad, some I fried, like the mushrooms, tomatoes, onions etc. The sweet potato slices were roasted with the sea bass, then I made up a salad of things I like, also a dressing or lemon and real honey.

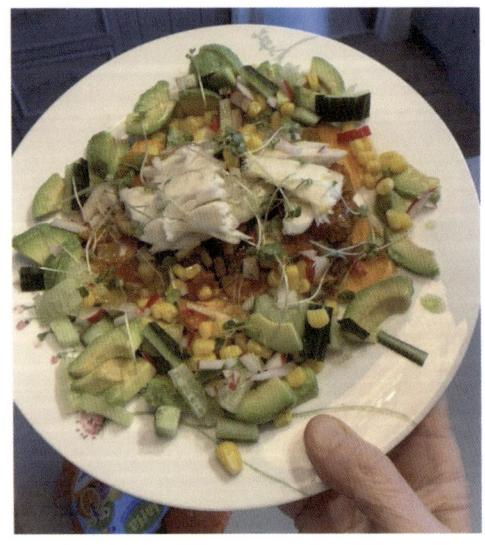 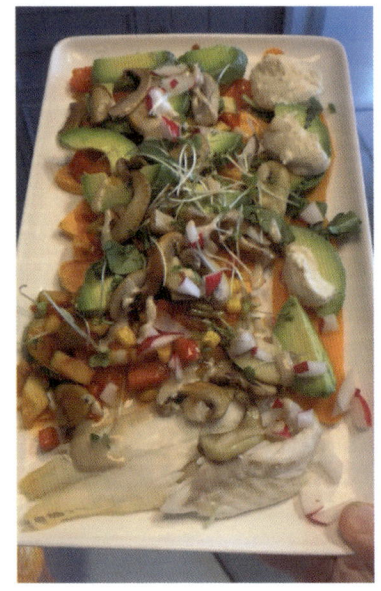

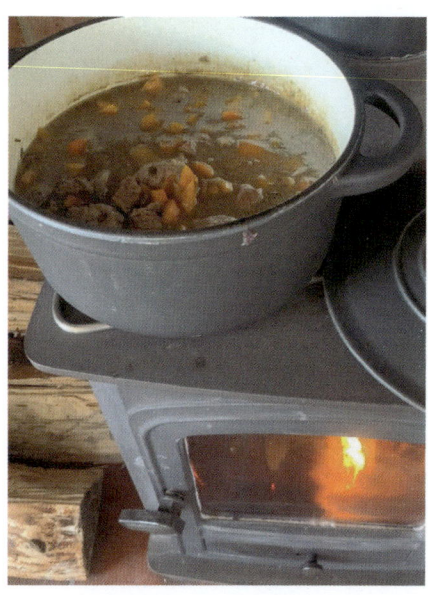 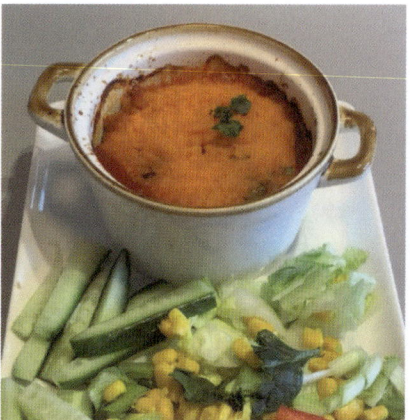 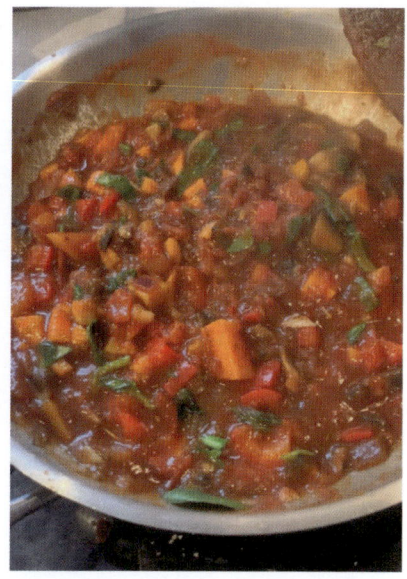

Hot pot and slow cookers can be very handy. I sometimes use our wood burner to cook meals on as it saves electric, and the cast iron pot makes everything taste nice. There have also been a few times when the electric has been off for various reasons. Casseroles in the oven are good as well. I add lots of veg and fresh herbs and buy meat from the butchers. The fats here aid gut healing.

I also have vegan hot pots, like this tomato and mushroom based one, with added, harissa, garlic. These are warming nutritious healthy meals for the winter, and easy to add spices and herbs and roots to, like, garlic, ginger and turmeric. Root veg is a super comfort food and easier to digest than rice, or pasta. The fibre in veg is better absorbed then grains.

This one is a tray bake, fresh herbs, a little water and olive oil, with added cabbage etc.

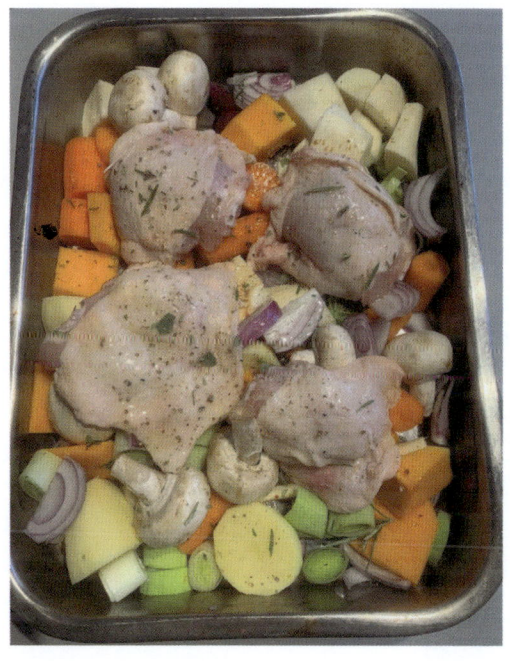 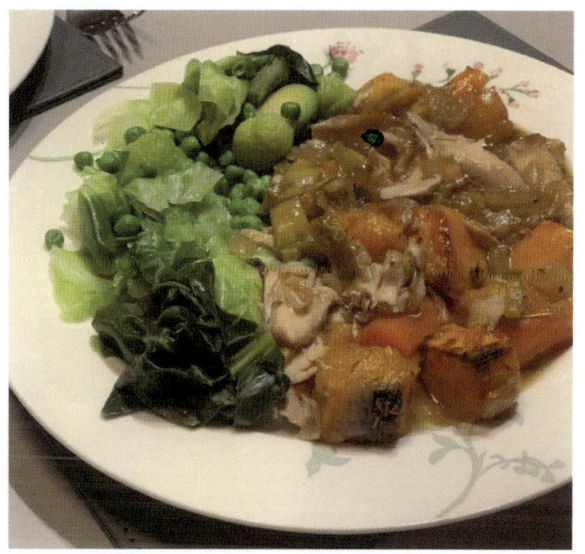

We could have this with prawns or salmon or cold turkey etc. I am happy with just this. These hot and cold mixed meals are good even in winter, when sometimes we don't wish a cold salad meal. Very little oils of fats are used and always a homemade dressing of olive oil, real honey and lemon, with either mustard, or garlic and added herbs of choice. Parsley, coriander, basil, etc.

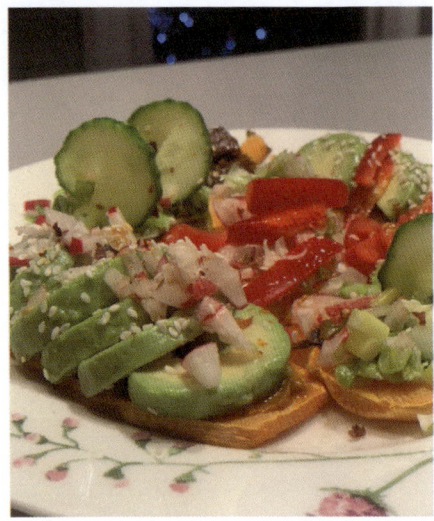
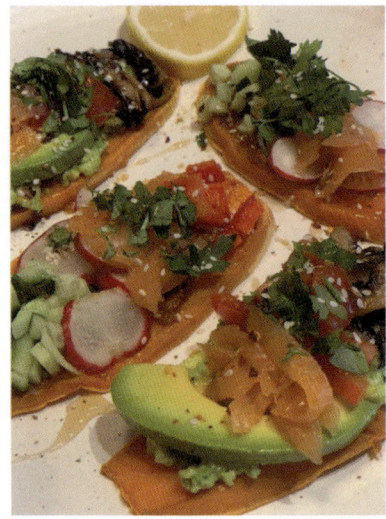

This meal is high in nutrition and very healing. The sweet potato is grilled and then the avocado is sliced on top with various salad items. We could add a little turkey or salmon. I like it on it's own. These sorts of meals are all helping heal the gut issues you maybe suffer with. As weaning off dairy, sugar, grains and eggs will all allow the gut to heal. I could of added cold turkey or beef, or prawns.

Alkaline and acids PH. Our bodies blood is slightly alkaline and needs to keep this way. If the balance becomes too acid, then our body will try to find alkaline minerals to buffer the imbalance and if this imbalance goes on long enough, it can take minerals from elsewhere, and calcium is an alkaline mineral. So, this shortage can mean losing bone mass, if the imbalance goes on for a very long time. So, eating lots of fresh and raw living foods, lightly cooked, over meats, grains, eggs, dairy, etc. Keeps this balance and our bodies happy, and our kidneys especially. As an acid body is a hot, inflamed burning body, where-as an alkaline body is a calm, cool contented body. Eating healthy foods helps keep our bodies in balance. People can and do heal on carnivore diets, but over a long time the high protein may impair the kidneys function, [there is science to say this] and the high fat also may cause problems. Meats are not cleansing, I believe people heal not because of the meats, but because they are avoiding the foods and drinks that cause problems. This is also the same for plant based diets, they heal because of what is avoided, more than the actual fruit and veg. But each to their own, there are many roads to Rome.

Acid and Alkaline balance

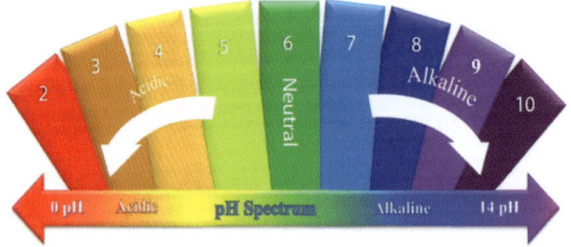

Snacks and sweet treats and puddings

We all love sweet treats, as our cells run on glucose which is a sugar. The trouble today is sugar is added into everything from ice cream, mint sauce, pasta sauces, stir fry sauces, cereals etc. now we have the sugar free products, which have sweeteners in them in place of sugar, which because they are chemically man made, our bodies and especially our livers don't know how to process them. So many puddings now are super unhealthy with all they add in to make us buy them. Going back to homemade puddings and eating them at least ¾ an hour after our main meal is best. Try to not have a pudding every day. If we have enough carbohydrates we will crave less sugar. Natural sugar in fruit is fine, we have been told now to fear too much fruit. There are many things I would fear before fruit, things like dairy, sugar, pork products, high fat meals, eggs, coffee, alcohol, diet cokes, etc, but I never fear fruit.

My go to snacks are dark chocolate [85% an over] medjool dates and coconut flakes. I make many little treats using these items. Also, I use cashew butter, cacao, gluten free oats, gluten free rice Krispies.

These treats are easy to make. Swapping the usual biscuits and cakes over to homemade flapjacks and homemade biscuits, which have coconut oil in place of dairy, real maples syrup or real honey in place of sugar or sweeteners is needed on a healing journey. Refined sugar and chemical sweeteners are super unhealthy and need weaning off from. When we have enough fruit in our diet it helps our liver store energy for when needed. The adrenals also prefer natural sugars to artificial ones, it helps keep them calm. Coffee being the biggest stressor for our adrenals, which sit on top of our kidneys. Getting the balance right for us take some thought, as too much chocolate or cacao can hinder our progress of wanting to heal. These battles we all have, finding healthier swaps helps.

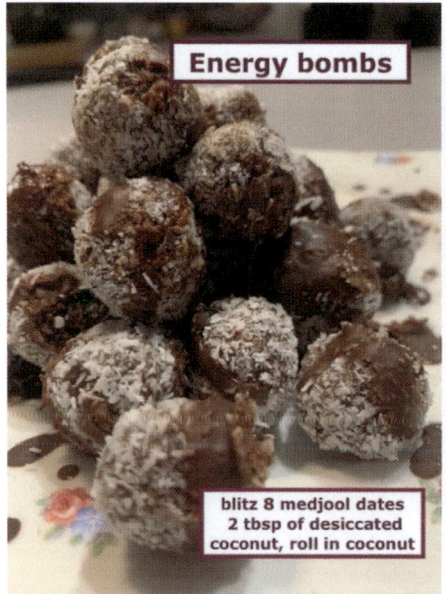

Energy bombs
blitz 8 medjool dates 2 tbsp of desiccated coconut, roll in coconut

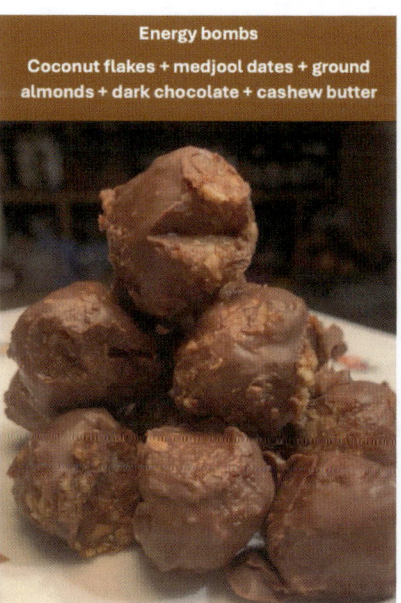

Energy bombs
Coconut flakes + medjool dates + ground almonds + dark chocolate + cashew butter

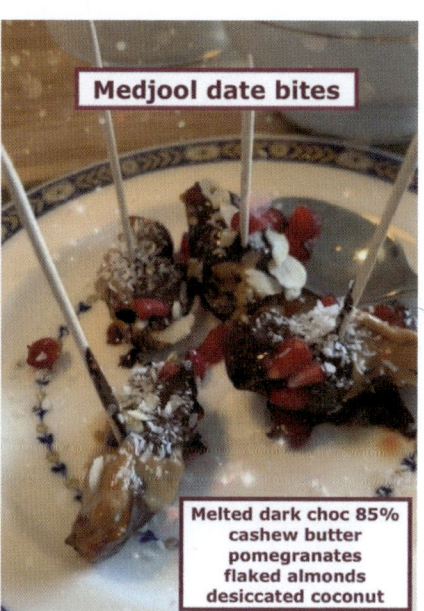

Medjool date bites
Melted dark choc 85% cashew butter pomegranates flaked almonds desiccated coconut

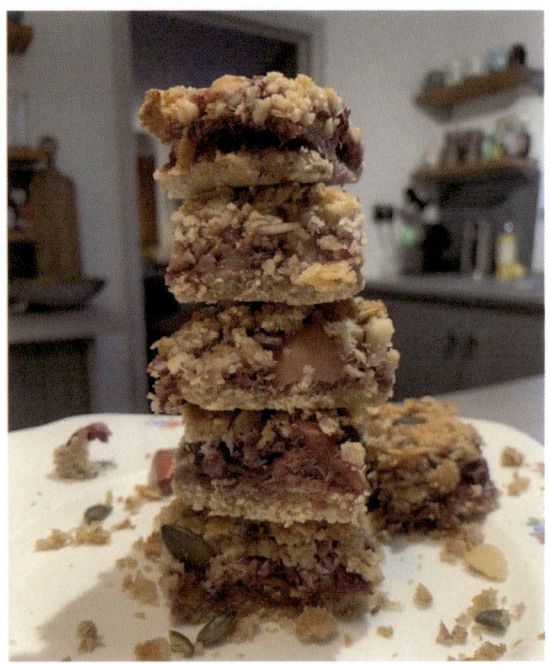
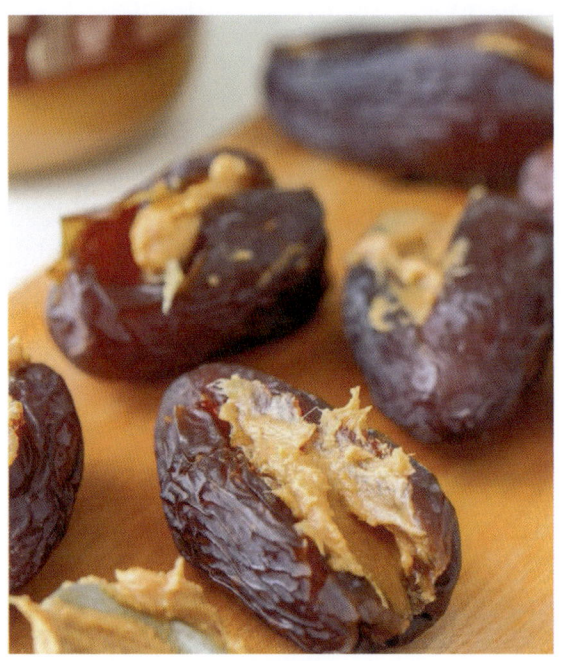

These crumble bars have no sugar in them, as I have used real maple syrup instead. It takes a little experimenting when we first start to swap out sugar, eggs and dairy and gluten, to get the amounts correct. My recipes are just a guide. As I am no great cook. Limiting sugar helps heal gut dysbiosis. I don't have puddings every day and if I need to adjust my weight or I am feeling sluggish, I would leave them out for a time. It's not about eating less, just better choices.

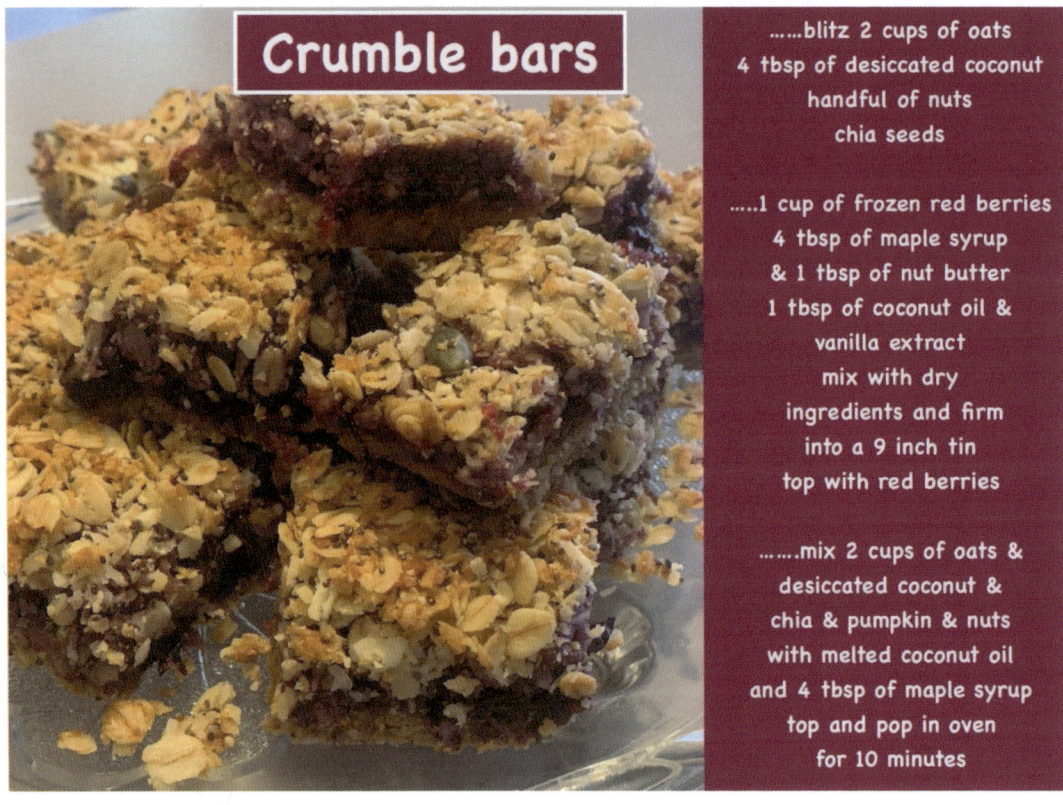

Crumble bars

……blitz 2 cups of oats
4 tbsp of desiccated coconut
handful of nuts
chia seeds

…..1 cup of frozen red berries
4 tbsp of maple syrup
& 1 tbsp of nut butter
1 tbsp of coconut oil &
vanilla extract
mix with dry
ingredients and firm
into a 9 inch tin
top with red berries

…….mix 2 cups of oats &
desiccated coconut &
chia & pumpkin & nuts
with melted coconut oil
and 4 tbsp of maple syrup
top and pop in oven
for 10 minutes

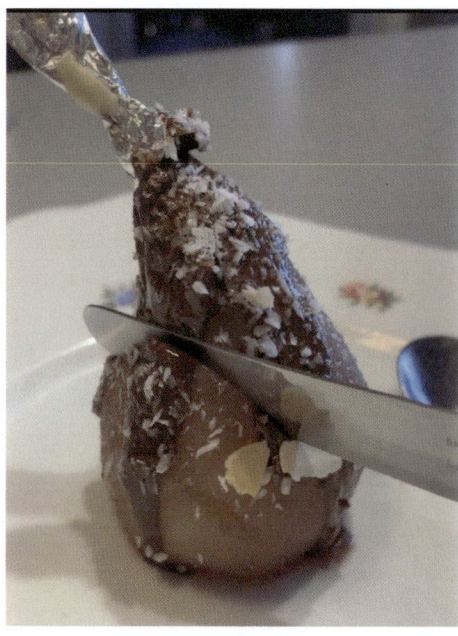 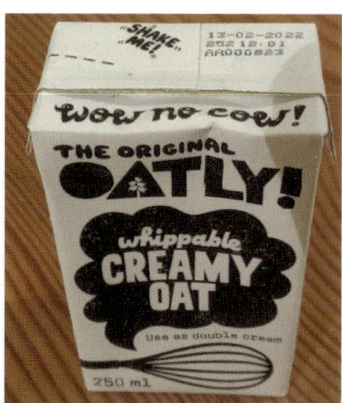 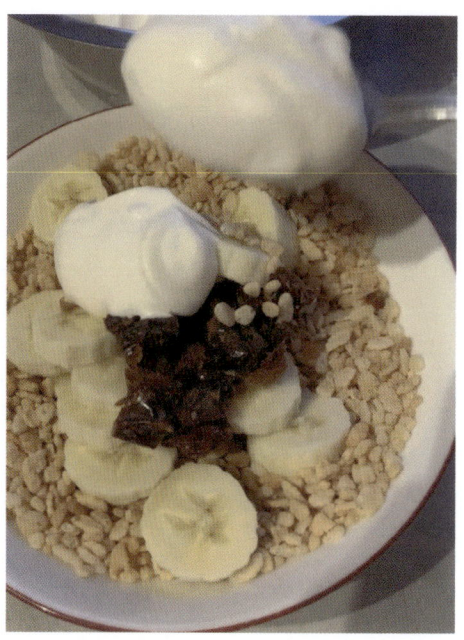

This pudding is poached pears in dark chocolate. The rice Krispies are gluten free, and I just added a banana, and a few cut up medjool dates, then I topped with Oatley whipping cream with a little added real maple syrup. The last one is fried bananas with Medjool's and real maples and again the whipping cream. These I don't have every day or even once a week. Its Christmas time as I am writing this book, so I have made these special occasion puddings as treats. I use flaked coconut for toppings.

This pudding is fried fruits in coconut oil, with a little Oatley/coconut cream and real honey.

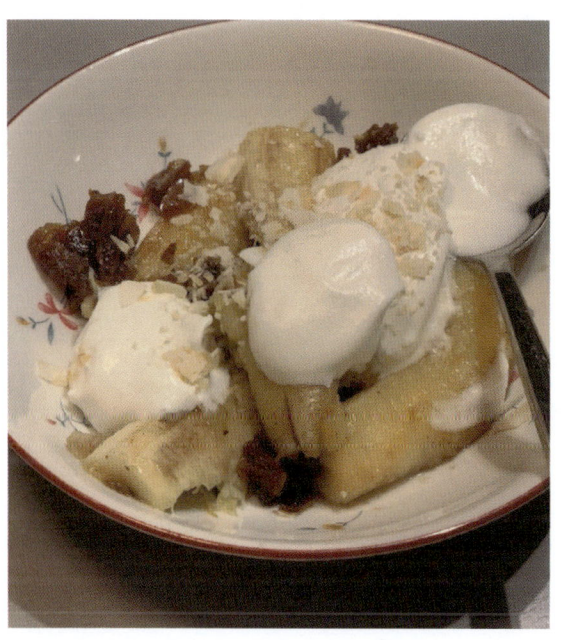 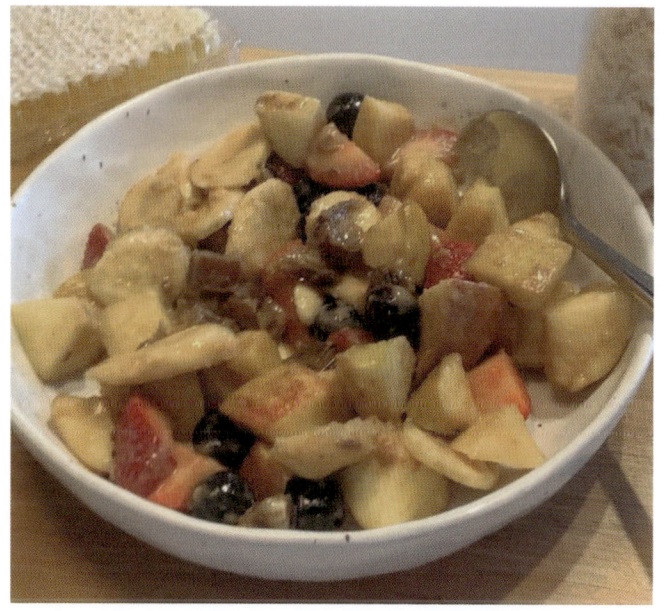

This crumble has no butter, I used coconut oil in its place. There is no sugar as I used real maples syrup, I swapped the cooking apples which are tart, so need more sweetness, for eating apples, the topping is oat flour, I blitzed myself, the red berry mix I used from frozen.

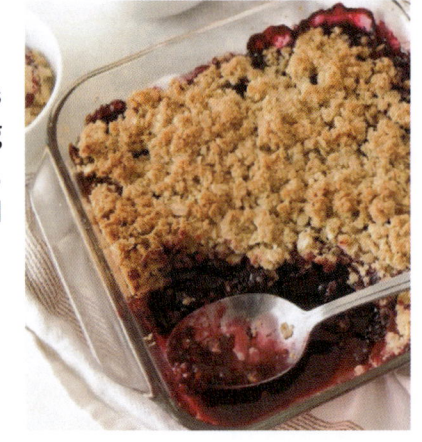

So, as you can see, it's easy to take a recipe form a magazine and adapt it, so it's a lot more healthy and avoids all the unhealthy ingredients.

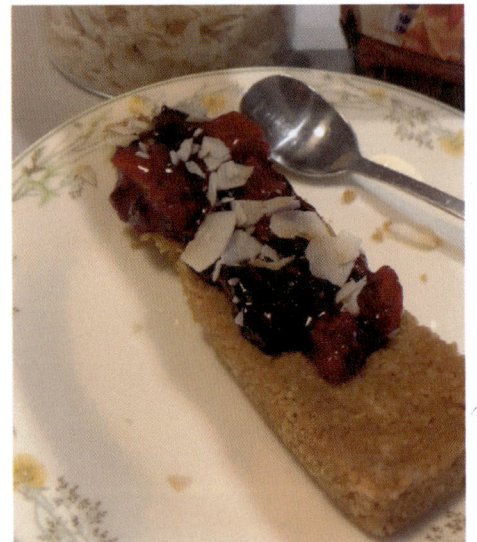

This biscuit is also one I have adapted and its made from blitzed gluten free rice Krispies. Experimenting to get the recipe right all takes time and practice, as learning new things always does, don't give up trying. There are many social media people sharing their healing journeys now. GF oats is another good biscuit maker.

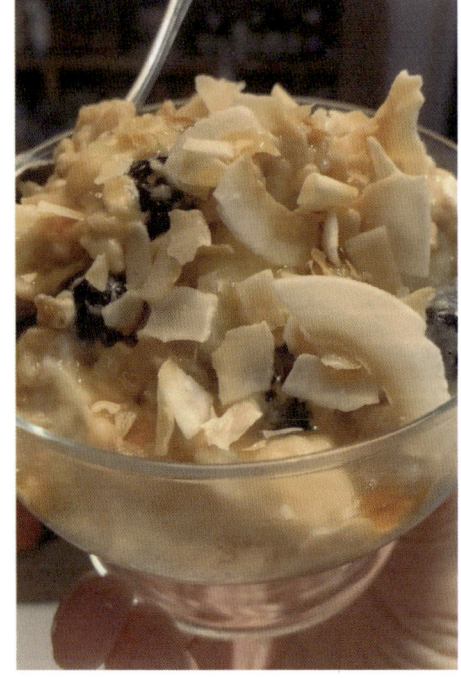

The banana pudding is fried banana with Cashew butter, medjool dates, blueberries, coconut oil, Oatley cream, [or coconut cream] dash of real maple syrup, GF rice Krispies and then topped with coconut flakes.

This trifle is a Christmas treat, it is dairy free, but not sugar free, as the custard and jelly will contain sugar and sweeteners, I would imagine. So not a pudding to have every week or even every month. Even though it has lots of fruit in it, that still doesn't make it a healing meal.

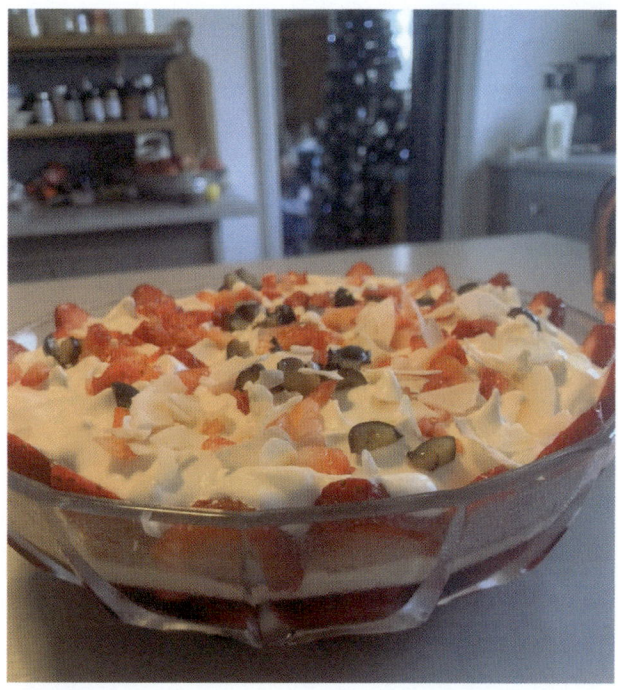

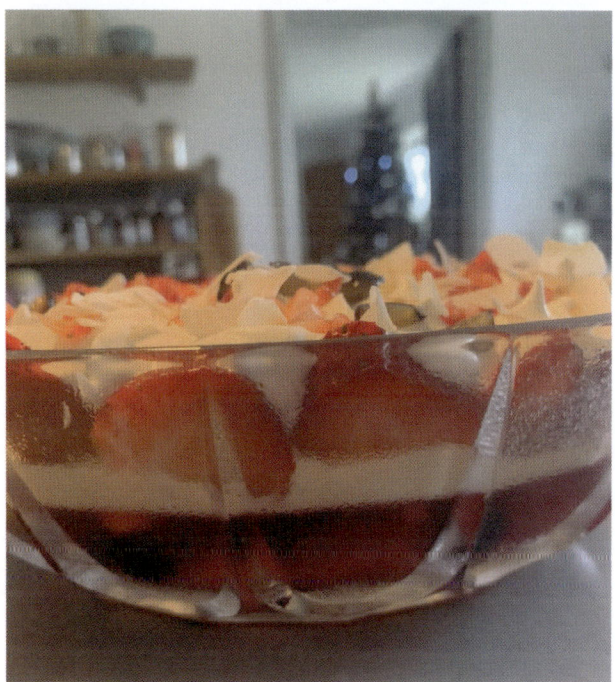

Try to choose things from the recipes and less of the problematic foods and drinks.
This is how we can slowly make improvements, by being mindful. We don't have to be 100% perfect, as long as we keep learning and improving each week and month.

Daily Healing Protocol for Chronic Health Conditions

Since many chronic health conditions share similar root causes, the protocols for healing are often alike. When I work with individuals, I tailor a specific protocol for their needs, so it can be beneficial to work with a local nutritionist or naturopath.

Best Start to the Day:
Lemon tea with warm water or ginger tea (add real honey or maple syrup if desired)

Healing Drinks:
Thyme tea (with or without honey)
Ginger tea with lemon (add honey or maple syrup if desired)
Ginger water, aloe vera water, coconut water
Hibiscus tea with honey or maple syrup, or other herbal teas (chamomile, mint, etc.)
Spices like cinnamon, nutmeg, ginger, and turmeric can be added to herbal teas
Cacao or dark chocolate, homemade hot chocolate, chicory drink, or coconut milk

Healing Juices:
Celery juice (top choice), or a blend of celery, cucumber, parsley, apples, and pears
Carrot, orange, ginger, and turmeric juice
Cucumber, apples, fennel, mint, or coriander juice (add herbs of choice)

Breakfast Options:
All fruits, smoothies (recipes in my book), melons, homemade apple or pear sauce with spices
Heavy metal detox smoothie
Gluten-free oats with red berries, mangoes, oranges, or bananas
Hot smoothies or apple/pear sauce with spices

Soups:
Roasted butternut squash, sweet potato, red pepper, mushroom, garlic, ginger, asparagus, peas, sweet potato, broccoli, cauliflower
Carrot and coriander soup

Healthy Snacks:
Medjool dates, nut butters (avoid peanut), fruits, salads, homemade sweet potato crisps
Dark chocolate (85% and above), homemade flapjacks, energy bombs, homemade fruit crumble with Oatley cream
Rice cakes, gluten-free crackers, homemade egg-free, dairy-free, gluten-free cakes or biscuits
Homemade sweet potato wraps

Lunch Ideas:
Salad with asparagus, avocado, beetroot (not in vinegar), tomatoes, cucumber, radishes, lettuce, cooked sweet potatoes, mushrooms, smoked or cooked salmon, red peppers, spinach, pomegranates, flaked almonds, sesame seeds, sundried tomatoes, tofu, spring onions, and a homemade dressing (garlic, lemon, mustard, honey)
Soup, tray-baked vegetables, hot pot, smoothies, or juices

Dinner (Tea):
Baked dishes, salads, soups, juices, smoothies, jacket potatoes, sushi, homemade stir fry with a little rice
Sea bass, mackerel, salmon, cabbage, Brussels sprouts, mashed potato, carrots, butternut squash, sweet potatoes, lentils, parsnips, courgettes, cauliflower, celeriac, swede, mushrooms

Puddings:
Lynn's homemade fruit crumble (dairy-free, gluten-free, sugar-free) using eating apples
Coconut oil, real honey or maple syrup, Oatley cream
Stewed pears or apples with real honey or maple syrup, cloves, cinnamon, and nutmeg
Homemade oat cakes, crumble bars, dark chocolate (85%)

Meal Timing & Tips:
Start the day with liquids like juices, smoothies, and herbal teas, and save heavier meals and fats for later in the day.
If you wake up hungry, opt for something quick and nutritious—there's flexibility in meal timing.
Avoid eating a large meal right before bed, as digestion may not occur properly.
If you feel hungry or thirsty at night, you may not have eaten or drunk enough during the day—aim to eat more earlier in the day.
Planning and preparing meals in advance is crucial, as healthy options can be scarce when you're out. Fast food is often the only option.
When at home and not rushed, it's easier to make nourishing meals. Prioritize making time for your health in today's fast-paced world.

Super Healing Foods
Food has incredible functional abilities—it can hydrate, provide abundant nutrition, reduce inflammation, fight pathogens, remove toxins, calm the adrenals, support liver cleansing, and aid digestion. On a healing journey, these foods should be consumed in abundance, alongside rest and relaxation.
Raw foods, particularly in juices and smoothies, retain their full enzyme and nutrient content, making them powerful healing tools.

Category	Foods
Algae & Sea Vegetables	Spirulina, Atlantic dulse, Seaweeds (kelp, nori, wakame), Samphire, Barley grass juice powder
Fresh Herbs & Medicinal Plants	Coriander, Basil, Parsley, Rosemary, Sage, Thyme, Oregano, Astragalus, Ashwagandha, Chamomile, Lavender, Ginseng, Ginkgo, Echinacea, Peppermint, Fennel, Aloe vera, Lemon balm
Spices & Healing Roots	Cinnamon, Nutmeg, Star anise, Cardamom, Paprika, Clove, Black cumin, Black pepper, Turmeric, Dill, Chilli powder, Cayenne pepper
Leafy Greens & Cruciferous Vegetables	Brussels sprouts, Cabbage, Leeks, Cauliflower, Broccoli, Kale, Spinach, Asparagus, Lettuce, Celery, Artichoke, Courgette, Bok choy, Arugula, Green beans, Peas, Watercress, Sorrel, Mustard leaves, Collard greens, Dandelion leaves
Salad Vegetables	Cucumber, Tomato, Radish, Peppers, Beets, Onions, Lettuce
Root Vegetables	Butternut squash, sweet potato, White potato, Carrots, Celeriac, Parsnips, Onions
Healing Fruits	Melons, Grapes, Oranges, Tangerines, Apples, Pears, Strawberries, Blueberries, Peaches, Pineapples, Raspberries, Cherries, Mangoes, Sharon fruit, Apricots, Kiwi, Cranberries, Papaya, Coconuts, Plums, Pomegranates, Bananas, Guava, Medjool dates, Grapefruit, Mulberries, Figs, Red currants, Blackberries, Dragon fruit, Lemons, Limes, Passion fruit, Avocados, Goji berries
Healing Mushrooms	Chaga, Reishi, Lion's mane, Shiitake, Cordyceps
Healthy Fats & Oils	Coconut oil, Olive oil, Avocado oil [use sparingly]

Foods That Don't Support Healing

These foods can be gradually reduced or eliminated while healing to allow the body to recover more effectively.

Dairy Products

Cheese, milk, butter, yogurt, kefir—all lack fibre and may contain added salt, sugar, artificial chemicals, or sweeteners.

Dairy is high in fat and can contribute to congestion in the body.

Eggs

Can be binding and congesting.

High in fats, which may not support detoxification.

Grains

Bread, pasta, pastry, rice, wraps—these are difficult to digest, especially for the young and elderly.

Gluten in wheat triggers inflammation in most people.

They dehydrate the body and irritate the gut lining.

For those with chronic health conditions, grains do not support healing—root vegetables are a better alternative.

Sugar

Refined sugar is hidden in many supermarket foods and is highly inflammatory.

Always read labels to avoid added sugars.

Better alternatives: Real maple syrup and raw honey (used sparingly, especially for those with diabetes or weight concerns).

Beans & Legumes

Can be difficult to digest compared to vegetables and fruits.

Sticking with a vegetable-based diet is often best for healing.

Beverages to Avoid

Coffee, alcohol, fizzy drinks, squash, store-bought smoothies, and processed juices—all are not healing.

Nuts & Seeds

Can be hard to digest and may cause issues.

Milled nuts or nut butters are easier, but many nut butters contain added palm oils and preservatives.

Historically, nuts were seasonal, not consumed year-round as they are today.

Processed & Factory-Farmed Meats

Pork products (bacon, sausages, deli meats) are high in fat and contain additives.

Factory-farmed meats contain chemicals from what the animals are fed.

While some people find healing on a carnivore diet, they often improve due to eliminating processed foods rather than consuming meat itself.

Meat is harder to digest than fruits and vegetables.

Harmful Oils

Vegetable and seed oils (used in deep frying) are inflammatory and unhealthy.

Better alternatives: Olive oil and coconut oil (used sparingly).

Artificial & Processed Ingredients

GMOs, MSG, and artificial chemicals used in food production.

Takeaways, factory-made ready meals, and store-bought baked goods contain preservatives and additives designed to extend shelf life, making them best avoided.

The Path to Healing: Removing & Rebalancing
True healing isn't just about adding nutrients or remedies—it's equally about identifying what to remove and avoid. By eliminating harmful foods, we make space for the nutrients our bodies truly need, creating the conditions for recovery and renewal.

Understanding the Causes of Poor Health
Poor health isn't anyone's fault. Many factors contribute to imbalances, including diet, environmental toxins, and modern lifestyle habits. In today's world, we are constantly exposed to substances that increase the risk of illness. However, by learning how to rebalance and nurture our bodies and minds, we can reverse these effects.

Awareness in Daily Choices

Food: Focus on the healthiest section of the supermarket—fresh fruits and vegetables.
Personal Care Products: opt for natural alternatives instead of chemical-laden sprays, perfumes, and body products. Many conventional sprays can be inhaled into the lungs, allowing harmful chemicals to enter the bloodstream.

Daily Healing Practices

Healing requires daily commitment and focus. Break unhealthy habits and replace them with nourishing routines. Develop awareness of how your environment and choices impact your health.

A Guide to Reclaiming Your Health
This book is designed to provide answers and practical solutions. With the right tools and knowledge, you can take control of your health and begin your journey to wellness.

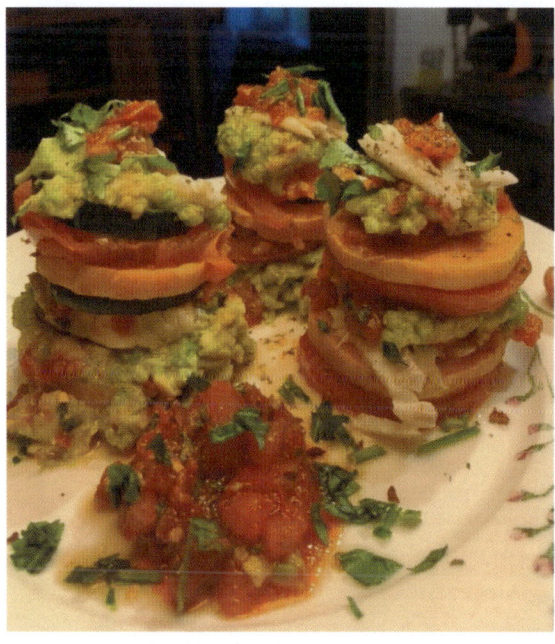
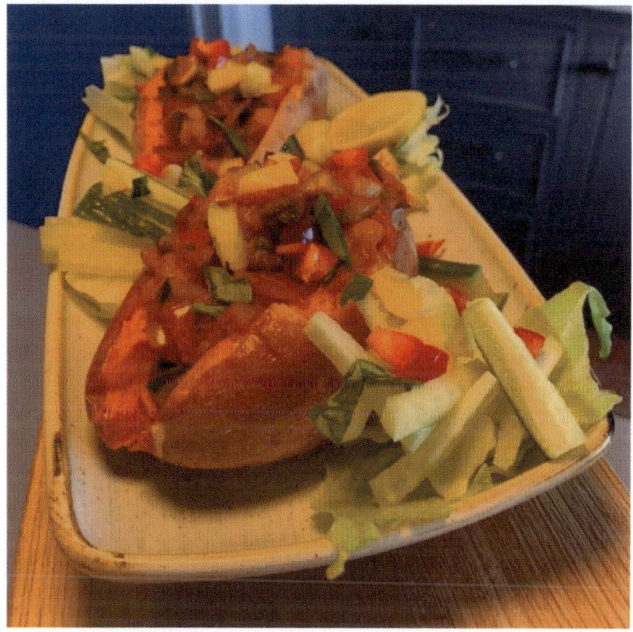

List of Chronic Conditions and Their Root Causes

As you can see, the same underlying factors contribute to many chronic health conditions. While this may seem overwhelming, it's actually a good thing—because it means that by addressing these root causes, we can create a single healing protocol that supports recovery across multiple conditions. By incorporating fresh herbs, spices, roots, juicing, and raw foods, we can provide the body with the nutrients it needs to restore balance and heal.

Scientific research on these conditions and their root causes can be found at **pubmed.com**

Neurological & Developmental Disorders

Autism, ADHD, Tourette's, Epilepsy, FND → Toxicity, heavy metals, gut dysbiosis, inflammation, poor liver detoxification, oxidative stress, redox imbalance

Respiratory Conditions

Asthma, COPD, Allergies → Congestion, inflammation, toxins, pathogens, viral infections (COPD), gut microbiome imbalances, heavy metals, chemical exposure, poor liver detox, redox imbalance

Autoimmune Diseases

General Autoimmune Conditions → Pathogens, viruses, inflammation, gut dysbiosis, toxins, stress, pharmaceutical damage, heavy metals, chemicals, trauma

Thyroid Disorders, Lupus, Rheumatoid Arthritis, Fibromyalgia, Psoriasis → Autoimmune-related causes (same as above)

Neurodegenerative & Cognitive Disorders

Multiple Sclerosis (MS) → Viral pathogens, inflammation, toxicity, heavy metals, chemical exposure, oxidative stress

Alzheimer's Disease → Blood sugar imbalance, inflammation, toxins, aluminium, heavy metals, chemical exposure

ALS (Motor Neuron Disease) → Toxicity, heavy metals, inflammation, chemicals

Dementia → Blood sugar imbalance, toxicity, gut dysbiosis, inflammation, oxidative stress, medication damage, heavy metals

Parkinson's Disease → Toxicity, mercury, aluminium, gut dysbiosis, blood sugar issues, heavy metals, chemicals

Mental Health Conditions

Anxiety → HPA axis dysfunction, adrenal imbalances, gut microbiome disruption, stress, trauma, inflammation, dehydration

Bipolar Disorder, Depression, ADHD → Trauma, abuse, stress, childhood adversity, gut inflammation, oxidative stress, adrenal dysregulation, nervous system imbalance, brain inflammation

Schizophrenia → Trauma, stress, toxicity, pathogens, oxidative stress, gut dysbiosis

OCD → Toxicity (heavy metals), stress, trauma, pathogens, oxidative stress, inflammation

POTS (Postural Orthostatic Tachycardia Syndrome) → Nervous system dysregulation, gut dysbiosis, toxicity, inflammation

Digestive Disorders

Celiac Disease, SIBO (Small Intestinal Bacterial Overgrowth) → Gut dysbiosis, bacterial overgrowth, strep bacteria, inflammation, parasites, heavy metals, chemical exposure

Chronic Fatigue Syndrome (ME/CFS) → Viral pathogens, inflammation, oxidative stress, heavy metals, pharmaceutical damage

Cancer → Toxicity, viral pathogens, heavy metals, oxidative stress, inflammation, parasites

IBS, IBD (Ulcerative Colitis, Crohn's Disease) → Pathogens (viruses, bacteria), inflammation, gut dysbiosis, toxins

Liver & Gallbladder Issues → Stagnation, toxicity, pathogens, inflammation, oxidative stress

Kidney Disease → Pathogens, toxins, high fat/protein diet, dehydration, inflammation

Metabolic & Hormonal Conditions

Type 2 Diabetes → Blood sugar imbalance, congested liver, gut dysbiosis, inflammation, oxidative stress

Type 1 Diabetes → Viral pathogens, infections damaging the pancreas

High Cholesterol → Stagnant liver, pathogens, toxicity, high-fat diet, inflammation

High Blood Pressure → Dehydrated, thickened blood, liver congestion, toxicity, pathogens, inflammation

Menopause Symptoms → Stagnant liver, lymph congestion, adrenal dysregulation, blood sugar imbalance, gut dysbiosis, toxicity

Reproductive & Hormonal Conditions

Endometriosis, Fibroids, PCOS, PMS → Pathogens (bacteria, viruses), inflammation, oxidative stress, blood sugar imbalance, adrenal dysregulation, liver and lymph congestion, heavy metals, chemical exposure

Prostate Issues → Viral pathogens, dehydration, oxidative stress, inflammation, toxicity

Skin & Inflammatory Conditions

Eczema, Psoriasis → Toxins, oxidative stress, gut dysbiosis, inflammation, heavy metals, liver congestion

Fibromyalgia → Pathogens (viruses, bacteria), inflammation, parasites, heavy metals, oxidative stress

Varicose Veins → Stagnant liver, lymph congestion, dehydration, oxidative stress, pathogens, toxins, inflammation

Infections & Pathogenic Conditions

UTIs (Urinary Tract Infections) → Yeast overgrowth, dehydration, oxidative stress, inflammation

Parasites → Gut dysbiosis, infection

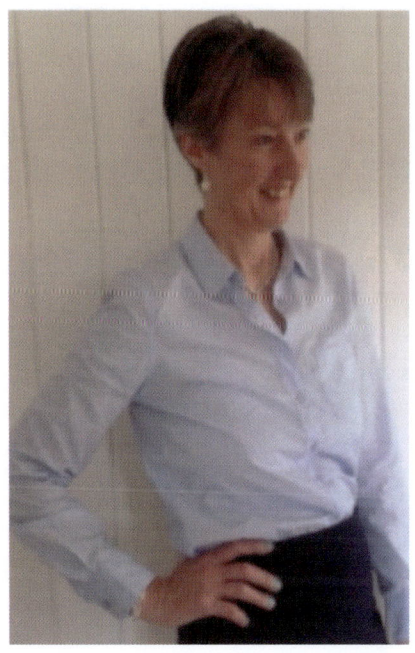

A Nutritional healing Guide to Reclaiming Your Health

This book is designed to offer answers, practical solutions, and actionable healing strategies. With the right knowledge, you can take **control of your health and begin your journey to wellness.**

Healing & Supplements

Holistic Healing Approaches:
- Nutrition & Detoxification – Nourish and cleanse the body with whole foods, fresh herbs, and natural remedies.
- Mind-Body Practices – Yoga, breathwork, sound healing (528 Hz), meditation, poetry, painting, journaling, and counselling.
- Physical Therapies – Massage, rebounding, handstand yoga stool, sauna, steam therapy, swimming, and walking.
- Environmental & Lifestyle Changes – Consider changing your job, home, or relationships if they negatively impact health.
- Self-Care Rituals – Essential oil diffusers, detox baths, castor oil packs, hydration, proper rest, relaxation, and quality sleep.
- Balanced Eating Habits – Eat and drink little and often to support digestion and energy levels.

Key Supplements & Superfoods
- Essential Vitamins & Minerals – Vitamin C, D, B12, zinc, omega-3s, and magnesium.
- Powerful Herbs & Adaptogens – Lemon balm, goldenseal, chaga mushrooms, turmeric, ginger, garlic, echinacea, elderberry, ginseng, ashwagandha, and cat's claw.
- Detox & Immune Support – Spirulina, barley grass juice powder, Atlantic dulse, black walnut hulls, oregano oil, milk thistle, and digestive enzymes.
- Antioxidants & Cellular Support – Astaxanthin, rose hip, Q10, NAC (N-acetyl cysteine), glutathione, L-lysine, and GABA.
- Healing Oils & Natural Remedies – Black seed oil, CBD oil, kelp, liquorice, hibiscus tea, chamomile tea, and real honey/maple syrup.

Best Cleansing & Detoxifying Foods

Incorporate fresh, hydrating, and anti-inflammatory foods into your daily routine through juices, smoothies, salads, soups, and steamed vegetables:
- Vegetables – Asparagus, cabbage, broccoli, sprouts, cauliflower, fennel, spinach, kale, celery, carrots, beetroot, onions, radishes, bell peppers, celeriac, and artichokes.
- Fruits – Pineapple, apples, pears, watermelon, pomegranate, lemons, limes, kiwi, mango, papaya, peaches, grapes, cherries, bananas, apricots, strawberries, raspberries, and blueberries.

Foods That Create Congestion & Mucus

These foods contribute to inflammation, stagnation, and toxicity in the body:
- Dairy – Cheese, milk, yogurt, ice cream.
- Grains – Bread, pasta, rice, pastry.
- Animal Products – All meats (especially processed meats), eggs.
- High-Fat & Processed Foods – Deep-fried foods, sugar, jams, jellies, fizzy drinks, caffeine, alcohol, fast food (lasagna, pizza, burgers, chips, omelettes, sausages, bacon, etc.).

Foods & Substances to Gradually Wean Off
If you're on a healing journey, consider slowly eliminating these over time:
- Inflammatory Foods – Eggs, dairy, grains, sugar, sweeteners, alcohol, coffee, black tea.
- Ultra-Processed Foods – Canned, jarred, packaged, and factory-made foods.
- Toxic Additives – MSG, GMOs, preservatives, artificial sweeteners, E-numbers.
- Fermented & Acidic Foods – Vinegar, pickled foods, and fermented products.

For optimal healing, focus on ancestral diets rich in alkaline, enzyme-rich foods—simple, whole, and unprocessed meals.

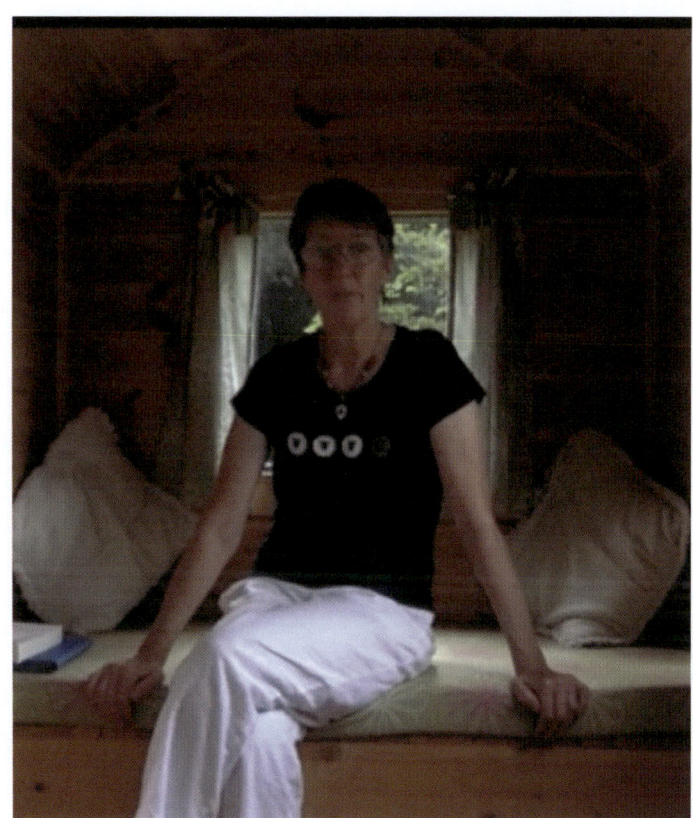

Sound healing frequencies to listen to. Or using weighted tunning forks on the body.

🌟Crown Chakra: 172.06 Hertz, deals with pure cosmic energy and is blocked by earthly attachments.
Enlightenment.

🌟Third Eye Chakra: 221.23 Hertz, deals with insight and is blocked by illusion. Return to spirituality.

🌟Throat Chakra: 141.27 Hertz, deals with truth and is blocked by lies. Awakening our intuition/instincts .

🌟Heart Chakra: 136.10 Hertz, deals with love and is blocked by grief. Connection and relationships.

🌟Solar Plexus Chakra: 126.22 Hertz, deals with will power and is blocked by shame. Transformation and miracles.

🌟Sacral Chakra: 210.42 Hertz, deals with pleasure and is blocked by guilt. Facilitating change.

🌟Root Chakra: 194.18 Hertz, deals with survival and is blocked by fear. Liberating guilt and fears.

Sound healing, relaxation, Yoga, walking, swimming and rest are all important healing modalities. That need practice.

432hz ALCHEMICAL CHAKRA ZODIAC CHART

Chakra	Frequencies	Purpose
CROWN CHAKRA (SAHASRARA)	A-108.00Hz / A-216.00Hz / A-432.00Hz / A-863.33Hz COAGULATION / CONSCIOUSNESS / KRONOS / UNDERSTANDING	Higher Wisdom Enlightenment (Thursday) SACHIEL
3RD EYE CHAKRA (AJNA)	D-144.00Hz / D-288.33Hz / D-576.00Hz / D-1155.00Hz DISTILLATION / THOUGHT / ZEUS / WISDOM	Returning to Spirituality (Saturday) CAFFIEL
THROAT CHAKRA (VISHUDDHA)	G-192.66Hz / G-384.66Hz / G-768.99Hz / G-1540.00Hz FERMENTATION / HEARING / ARIES / SEVERITY	Awakening Intuition (Wednesday) RAPHAEL
HEART CHAKRA (ANAHATA)	C-128.33Hz / C-257.00Hz / C-514.00Hz / C-1028.00Hz CONJUNCTION / TOUCH / HELIOS / BEAUTY	Connection and Relationships (Monday) GABRIEL
SOLAR PLEXUS CHAKRA (MANIPURA)	F#-181.66Hz / F#-363.66Hz / F#-726.66Hz / F#-1452.00Hz SEPARATION / SIGHT / APHRODITE / MERCY	Transformation and Miracles (Sunday) MICHAEL
SACRAL CHAKRA (SVADHISTHANA)	Eb-152.66Hz / Eb-305.33Hz / Eb-611.33Hz / Eb-1221.00Hz DISSOLUTION / TASTE / HERMES / GLORY	Facilitating Change (Friday) ANAEL
ROOT CHAKRA (MULADHARA)	Bb-114.33Hz / Bb-229.00Hz / Bb-457.33Hz / Bb-915.00Hz CALCINATION / SMELL / LUNA / FOUNDATION	Liberating Guilt and Fear (Tuesday) CAMAEL

References
On my journey I have found many helpful people online to guide me in my choices as I was trying desperately to heal. Here are some of the most helpful people I found on my own healing journey. Pubmed.com is a great resource to start learning about health and conditions.
Medicalmedium.com. Anthony William
Doctors David Jockers
Robert Morse ND
Amy Myers MD
Mark Hyman MD
Always talk to your own doctor and keep up to date with all your health check-ups, blood tests and hospital visits regarding your own health. Nutrition is not a medical replacement.

Researching any particular condition on **pubmed.com** is a fantastic way to deepen your understanding of illness! 🧠💡 Simply type in keywords like **"lupus"** or **"endometriosis"** alongside terms such as **"oxidative stress"**, and you'll uncover **hundreds—if not thousands—of studies**. 📚🔍

From there, you can **select key studies** to build a clearer picture of the condition and potential healing strategies. This approach helps us **gather crucial information** to create a **bespoke health plan** tailored to our unique needs. ✨📝

As I've mentioned before, many **chronic illnesses share common root causes**—including **pathogens, parasites, depleted nutrition, oxidative stress, viruses, and Mold.** 🦠⚡ To truly heal, we must **address all these factors daily** through **a well-designed nutritional plan.** 🍏🥦 Over time, the goal is to **refine our choices** until we reach a level that supports deep healing and lasting wellness. 🌿💪

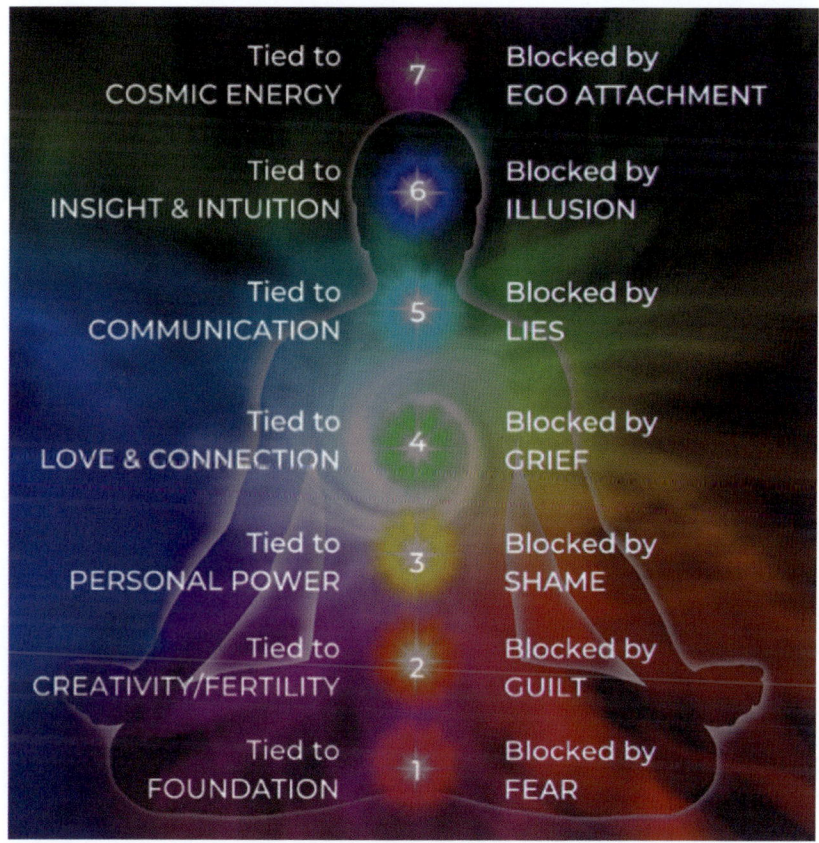

Colds and flu, sore throats and coughs...

🌬️🤧 Do we catch a cold, or do we create one? A bit of both, I think! If we're stressed, overworked, and neglecting rest, our immune system takes a hit. 😴⚡ Without enough sleep and relaxation, we become more vulnerable to illness.

🛡️ Building and restoring our immune system requires nutrient-rich foods, fresh herbs, spices, and powerful roots like ginger, garlic, and turmeric. 🥕🧄🌿 One of my go-to remedies is a healing broth—I make it ahead of winter, strain it, and freeze it alongside some homemade elderberry syrup. ❄️🍇

🚑 Whenever someone in my family starts feeling under the weather—a cough, sore throat, or cold—I quickly heat up the broth, and they sip it throughout the day. ☕🔥 This is true healing.

💊 These days, many rush to the pharmacy, spending a small fortune on suppressant drugs. 💊💰 But these often block the body's natural detox process, stopping it from clearing out mucus and pathogens. 🤢❌ Instead, we should hydrate well and allow our bodies to burn the virus out naturally. 💦🔥

🏥 Of course, if we become seriously ill, a doctor or hospital may be necessary. But there's so much fear around our own bodies now. Many no longer trust their immune systems. Once we focus on deep healing and rebuilding health, we gain faith in our body's resilience. 💪🌟

🛠️ Health and healing require effort—but when we work with our bodies, not against them, the rewards are life-changing. ❤️✨

🌶️ We all experience illness from time to time—fevers, upset stomachs, or loss of appetite. During these times, it's best to give the digestive system a break and stick to homemade juices, herbal broths, or spicy soups. 🍲 Resting, staying warm, and keeping hydrated all help the body heal faster. 🛏️💧

🌀 Extra immune boosters to speed up recovery:

🌿 Steam inhalations with eucalyptus oil 🌱💨

💊 Immune-supporting supplements like garlic, ginger, turmeric, echinacea, + buffered vitamin C

☀️ Vitamin D in winter for immune support

🍵 Herbal teas like thyme and elderberry to soothe the throat and fight viruses

🍍 Pineapple as a natural throat soother

🍯 Real honey, lemon balm, and zinc lozenges for extra healing

🧂 Gargling with salt water to cleanse the throat

🚫 What to avoid while healing:

❌ Dairy 🥛, eggs 🥚, meat 🥩, milk chocolate 🍫

❌ Alcohol 🍷, coffee ☕, grains 🌾, cake 🍰, sugar 🍬

❌ Processed meats like bacon and sausages

🍎 Easy-to-digest foods like apple or pear sauce provide energy while being gentle on the stomach. Spices, roots, and fresh herbs all work in harmony to help the body recover. 🌿✨

💦 Hydration is key—flush out toxins and support your body's natural healing process! 🚰🔥

🥣✨ Immune-Boosting Healing Broth ✨🥣

🧅 **Vegetables:** 🧅 1 onion + 1 leek + 🥕 3 carrots + 🌿 3 stalks of celery + 🍅 4 tomatoes

🌿 **Herbs:** 🌿 ¼ tsp rosemary + ¼ tsp sage + ¼ tsp thyme + ¼ tsp parsley + ¼ tsp coriander + ¼ tsp oregano

🌶️ **Spices & Roots:** 🧂 ¼ tsp cinnamon + ¼ tsp turmeric + ½ tsp ginger + ¼ tsp cumin + ¼ tsp nutmeg + ⭐ 2 star anise + ¼ tsp fennel + 5 cloves + 5 cardamom pods + 🌶️ Shake of cayenne pepper + 🖤 Shake of black pepper

🧄 **Extras for Immune Power:** 🧄 1 whole bulb of garlic + 🍄 1 cup of shiitake mushrooms + 🍯 A drizzle of real honey

🌊 **Liquid Base:** 💦 3 pints of water

🍊 **Citrus Boost:** 🍊 ¼ orange + 🍋 ¼ lemon

🌿 **Finishing Touches:** 🌿 3 bay leaves + 🧂 Himalayan salt to taste

🔥 **Instructions:** 1 Add all ingredients to a large pot. 2 Bring to a gentle simmer and let it cook for 2 hours. 3 Strain and sip throughout the day for deep nourishment and immune support. 💛✨

A powerhouse of healing herbs, spices, and nutrients to boost immunity, warm the body, and fight off infections naturally! 💪🍲🌿

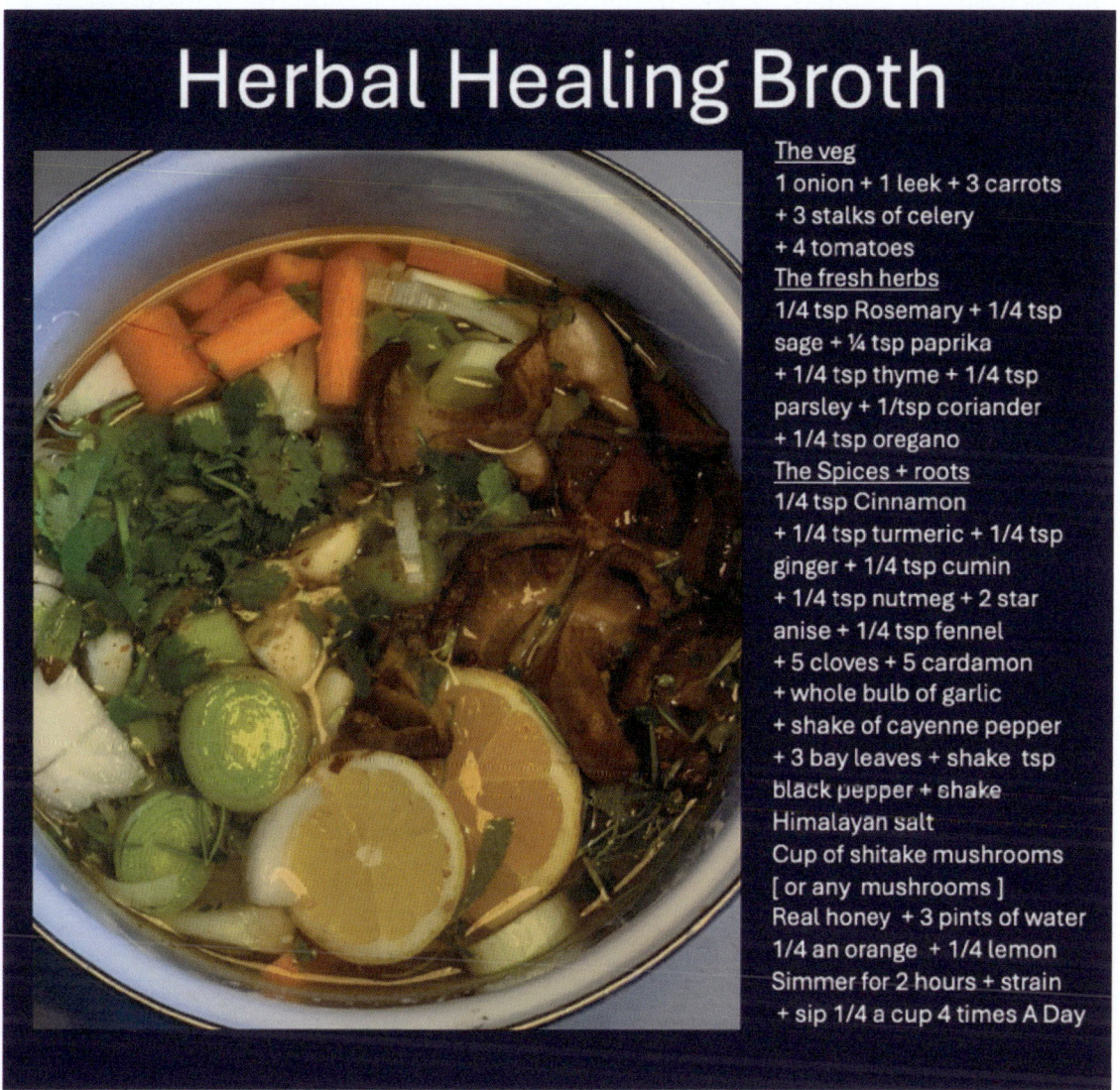

Herbal Healing Broth

The veg
1 onion + 1 leek + 3 carrots + 3 stalks of celery + 4 tomatoes

The fresh herbs
1/4 tsp Rosemary + 1/4 tsp sage + ¼ tsp paprika + 1/4 tsp thyme + 1/4 tsp parsley + 1/tsp coriander + 1/4 tsp oregano

The Spices + roots
1/4 tsp Cinnamon + 1/4 tsp turmeric + 1/4 tsp ginger + 1/4 tsp cumin + 1/4 tsp nutmeg + 2 star anise + 1/4 tsp fennel + 5 cloves + 5 cardamon + whole bulb of garlic + shake of cayenne pepper + 3 bay leaves + shake tsp black pepper + shake Himalayan salt
Cup of shitake mushrooms [or any mushrooms]
Real honey + 3 pints of water
1/4 an orange + 1/4 lemon
Simmer for 2 hours + strain + sip 1/4 a cup 4 times A Day

Healing Properties of the Herbs, Spices, and Ingredients in the Broth ✨

🌿 Vegetables

🧅 Onion – Antibacterial, antiviral, and supports respiratory health. Rich in sulphur compounds that boost immunity.

🌿 Leek – Supports gut health, high in prebiotic fibre, and aids detoxification.

🥕 Carrots – Rich in beta-carotene (Vitamin A) for immune support and eye health.

🌿 Celery – Anti-inflammatory, supports digestion, and helps flush out toxins.

🍅 Tomatoes – High in lycopene, a powerful antioxidant that supports heart and immune health.

🌿 Healing Herbs

🌿 Rosemary – Improves circulation, enhances memory, and has antimicrobial properties.

🌿 Sage – Supports cognitive function, soothes sore throats, and has antibacterial effects.

🌿 Thyme – Powerful antiviral and antibacterial properties; great for respiratory health.

🌿 Parsley – Rich in Vitamin C, supports kidney function, and detoxifies heavy metals.

🌿 Coriander (Cilantro) – Helps detox heavy metals, supports digestion, and is anti-inflammatory.

🌿 Oregano – Natural antibiotic, antiviral, and antifungal properties; supports gut health.

🌶️ Spices & Roots

🧂 Cinnamon – Regulates blood sugar, boosts circulation, and has antibacterial properties.

🌿 Turmeric – Strong anti-inflammatory and antioxidant; supports brain and immune health.

🧄 Ginger – Improves digestion, fights infections, and reduces inflammation.

🌿 Cumin – Aids digestion, supports detoxification, and is antimicrobial.

🌰 Nutmeg – Supports brain function, aids digestion, and has antibacterial properties.

⭐ Star Anise – Antiviral, supports respiratory health, and is used in flu remedies.

🌿 Fennel – Soothes digestion, reduces bloating, and supports liver detoxification.

🧄 Garlic – Natural antibiotic, antiviral, and antifungal; supports heart health.

🌶️ Cayenne Pepper – Boosts circulation, aids digestion, and clears mucus.

🖤 Black Pepper – Enhances nutrient absorption, especially for turmeric.

🧂 Himalayan Salt – Rich in minerals, helps hydration, and supports electrolyte balance.

🍄 Mushrooms & Other Superfoods

🍄 Shiitake Mushrooms – Boosts immune function, reduces inflammation, and supports gut health.

🍯 Real Honey – Antibacterial, antiviral, soothes sore throats, and supports wound healing.

🍊 Citrus Boost

🍊 Orange – High in Vitamin C, supports immune function, and fights oxidative stress.

🍋 Lemon – Alkalizing, detoxifying, and rich in Vitamin C for immunity.

🌿 Extras

🌿 Bay Leaves – Supports digestion, antimicrobial, and helps clear congestion.

This broth is a powerful healing elixir, loaded with immune-boosting, anti-inflammatory, and detoxifying properties — for fighting colds, flu, and infections while nourishing the body! 💪🍲✨

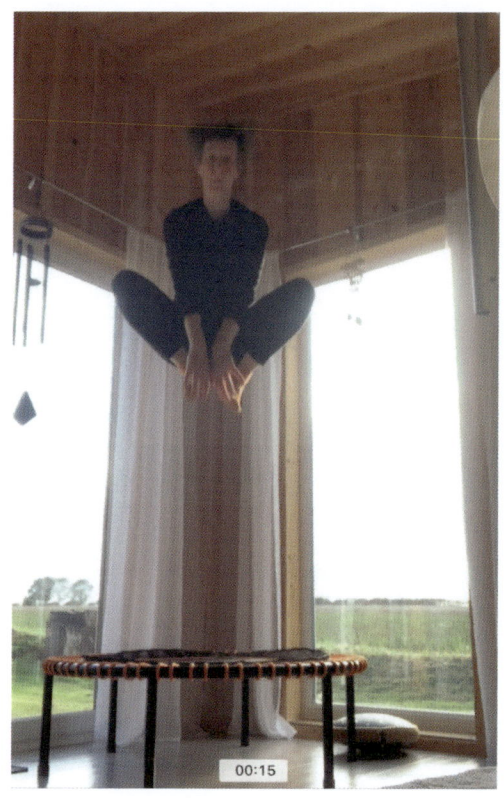 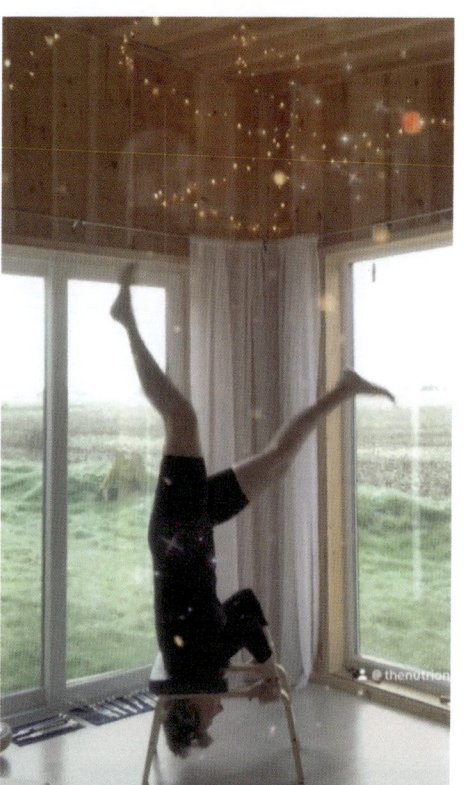

Exercise aids healing, but don't overdo it, gentle walking, swimming or Yoga is fine. I like rebounding and it's a great way to get the lymphatic system moving. This trampoline is a Bellicon make, which are the best, they have bungees ropes to your weight and softer on the knees. Some have springs which are hard on the joints. I bought this second hand and added new bungees. So, it's like new now.

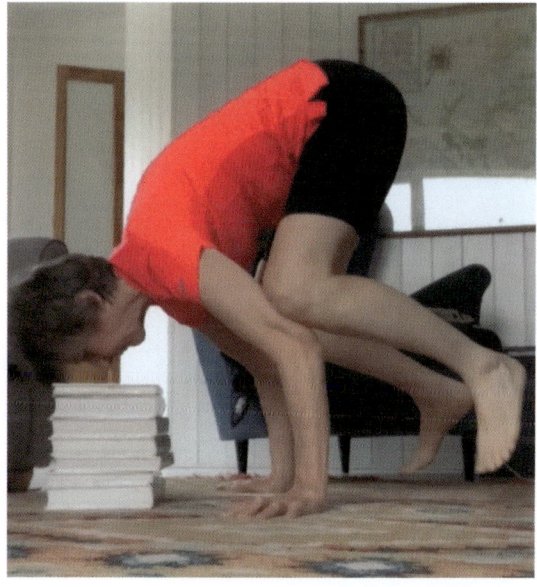

I hope you are inspired to start your healing journey and can find enough healthy lovely recipes to try.

Printed in Great Britain
by Amazon